W9-DFD-531

Landscape Painting with Markers

Landscape Painting with Markers

By Harry Borgman

WATSON-GUPTILL PUBLICATIONS, NEW YORK

PITMAN PUBLISHING, LONDON

Copyright © 1977 by Watson-Guptill Publications

First published 1977 in the United States and Canada by Watson-Guptill Publications,
a division of Billboard Publications, Inc.,
1515 Broadway, New York, N.Y. 10036

Library of Congress Cataloging in Publication Data
Borgman, Harry.
   Landscape painting with markers.
   1. Landscape in art. 2. Dry marker drawing—
Technique. I. Title.
NC878.B67 1977   743′.8′36   77-9345
ISBN 0-8230-2635-3

Published in Great Britain by Pitman Publishing Ltd.,
39 Parker Street, London WC2B 5PB
ISBN 0-273-01148-1

All rights reserved. No part of this publication may be
reproduced or used in any form or by any means—graphic,
electronic, or mechanical, including photocopying, recording,
taping, or information storage and retrieval systems—
without written permission of the publishers.

Manufactured in U.S.A.

First Printing, 1977

To James H. Donahue

Contents

Introduction

MARKERS ARE versatile instruments: they are premixed, ready for instant use, have an endless color range, dry instantly, and are compatible with most painting surfaces. Furthermore, the colors are transparent, and, even with a limited palette, a great variety of colors can be created by using one color over another. Markers offer a fast, convenient way to do sketches and paintings with a minimum of equipment. Brushes, waterbowls, mixing trays, and the eventual cleanup that accompanies these materials are eliminated.

This sounds like a wonder medium, doesn't it? Well, many people think it is. Because of the ease of use and the tremendous range of available colors, the popularity of markers has grown a great deal. It's hard to find a more ideal medium for sketching, drawing, or painting. Markers are especially well-suited for doing preliminary sketches to use later as references for paintings done in other mediums.

Because of the rather extensive range of colors, you may be confused when you begin to choose a palette. Some brands not only feature primary and secondary colors, but middle-tone values and pastel hues as well. I recommend the basic color palette shown on page 113. You can start out with this basic palette and gradually change it to suit your needs as you develop.

In the first chapter of this book, I will tell you about the different marker brands available and demonstrate the various marks that can be made with the different nibs. In Chapter 2, many marker techniques done on various paper surfaces are shown, including how pens and pencils can be used in conjunction with markers. In the later chapters, many subjects, including trees, grasses, water, snow, mountains, skies, clouds, and architecture, are detailed in separate chapters through step-by-step demonstrations. Included are several color demonstrations showing various color techniques. It would be a good idea to copy all of these concise step-by-step demonstrations as exercises when practicing with markers. If you do this as a beginner, you will gain knowledge of marker techniques and a firm foundation from which to grow. If you are a graphic artist or illustrator and you are already using markers in your work, perhaps you will find a new technique or rendering idea. If you are an art school instructor, you will be able to use many of the exercises and demonstrations as the basis for class assignments.

But remember—whether you are a beginner, a graphic artist, a teacher, or a student—to develop yourself fully in this medium, you must devote a certain amount of time to practicing. This is not a skill that can be learned at one sitting—you must practice constantly and learn the advantages and limitations of this technique.

A WORD OF CAUTION ABOUT MARKERS

Many nonwaterbased markers contain dyes, resins, and organic solvents. Different brands use different solvents, and many of them are dangerous. At this time, although the hazards of a number of the dyes are not known, aromatic hydrocarbons, such as xylol and toluol, are definitely dangerous. Read the labels on the markers very carefully. Young children should never be allowed to use these types of markers because of their susceptibility to the effects of organic solvents. For people of all ages, adequate ventilation is necessary when working with nonwaterbased markers. Open windows or an exhaust fan are highly recommended. It's also a good idea to wear gloves when handling the nibs directly or to hold them with pliers.

CHAPTER ONE

Materials and Equipment

MARKERS HAVE gained tremendously in popularity over the last few years. There are quite a few brands available, and these come in all kinds of shapes and sizes, many brands offering an extensive color selection. Choosing a brand of markers is largely a personal matter. I would suggest checking out the available brands in your local artist supply store and buying three or four types that feel right in your hand. You can work with these at home and then make your decision. Be sure to check out the color charts of the various brands to see how extensive they are.

There are basically two types of markers: the permanent oil base, waterproof type, and the water soluble type. The nibs come in a variety of sizes and shapes, ranging from extra large and broad to medium, fine, and extra fine. The nibs are shaped in chisel, square, round, bullet, and pencil form. Many of them are made of felt, while others consist of nylon or other plastic materials. The marker colors themselves are dyes, rather than pigments, and have a tendency to fade over a long period of time or when exposed to sunlight. Markers must be capped tightly after use to prevent the dye from drying out.

The fine-line markers are excellent for all types of sketching, drawings, and even lettering. The broader ones are usually multifaceted—you can create a variety of line weights by drawing with the different edges.

Besides the markers themselves, the only other basic material you will need (besides a flat surface) is paper. Marker colors tend to saturate most papers, and the colors then are difficult to blend. However, rice papers—which are very absorbent—allow the colors to blend quite easily because the paper stays damp while you work on it. A hard, glossy surface enables you to rework areas as the dyes lay on the surface rather than penetrate underneath.

If you're a beginner, unfamiliar with markers, I suggest that you limit your first attempts to working in grays and black. Working in black and white is much simpler, making it easier for you to learn how to handle this medium. Color rendering is much more complex and should not be attempted until you have a thorough knowledge of what markers can and cannot do. After you feel at home with markers, then start working with color.

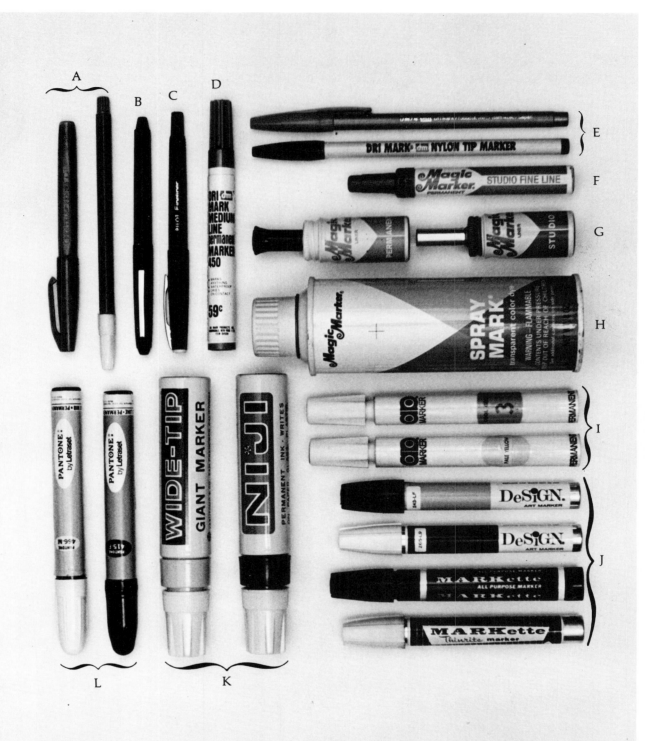

Markers come in all shapes and sizes—try a few different brands and see how they feel to work with before you decide to buy a complete set. Here are a few different kinds: (A) two different types from Pentel—the Pentel Sign Pen and the Pentel 67; (B) Niji Stylist; (C) Pilot Fineliner; (D) Dri Mark 450; (E) Dri Mark fine line pens; (F) Studio Fine Line by Magic Marker; (G) Studio Magic Markers; (H) Spray Mark by Magic Marker; (I) AD Markers; (J) pens by Eberhard Faber—the Design Art Marker, Markette All Purpose, and the Markette Thinrite; (K) Niji wide-tip giant; (L) Pantone by Letraset.

MARKERS

I have used most marker brands over the years and personally feel most comfortable with the Magic Marker Studio markers. I guess I've grown used to them and their color range. This is the first brand I remember seeing on the market, and I've used them for a long time. I work with markers a great deal in the commercial art field doing advertising layouts and television storyboards. I do most of this work with Magic Markers, although at times I use other fine brands, such as AD Markers, Design Art Markers, Prismacolor, and Pantone. Although all of these have an extensive color selection, Magic Markers have one advantage over the others—the screw-on cap and the inner fibrous core can easily be removed. This core, containing the marker dye, can be held with a pair of pliers (or gloves) and used to produce a very smooth, flat tone over a large area without difficulty.

Magic Marker Studio Markers. This is the brand I generally use. The colors flow smoothly through a unique 4-way broad, felt tip and dry instantly. They are waterproof, smudge proof, and never need fixing. Other markers also have these same qualities, but Magic Markers have one of the largest range of colors available (186). The markers are available individually, in sixteen 12-color sets, sets of 48, or a set of 150 with which a convenient wood tray is included.

Magic Markers are also available with a pointed nib for fine line work. These fine-line markers come in 70 colors, can be purchased individually or in 12-color sets, and match the Studio marker colors. They have color-coded caps and holders that allow for fast color identification.

Another interesting product from Magic Marker is the Spray Mark, transparent spray colors that can be used to cover large areas. The sprays come in 36 colors that are available separately or in three sets of 12 colors each. These colors are also coordinated with the Magic Marker Studio line. A great advantage of Spray Mark is that it can be used on any surface, including foil, glass, plastic, and metal, as well as paper.

AD Markers. These markers, which come with regular or fine-pointed nibs, are available in 18 sets of 12 permanent colors each. The large AD Marker Centurion set contains 19 grays, 17 reds, 16 blues, 12 yellows, 14 greens, and 22 browns, all in a redwood box. Three different point styles are available to replace the regular wedge-shaped tip on the standard marker.

Design Art Markers. Design Art Markers, by Eberhard Faber, come in a complete range of colors. The regular, broad chisel tip comes in 96 colors; the pointed and ultra-fine nibs come in 48 colors each. These markers can be purchased in 12-color sets as well as separately, and the Director's Assortment is a portable carousel of 72 regular, broad-tipped colors.

Dri Mark. Dri Mark produces a lower cost marker available in 36 colors in either nylon-tipped fine-line or medium-line versions.

Flo-Master. Flo-Master felt-tip pens are versatile drawing and painting instruments. There are eight different, wool felt nibs that can be used with the standard Flo-Master pen. These nibs come in fine, bullet, angled, chisel, and T-shapes. Also available is an oversized pen for greater ink capacity—these pens do not contain their own color supply and must be filled with inks or dyes. Eight transparent and five opaque Flo-Master colors are available in convenient containers with spouts. You can mix your own colors, with these—

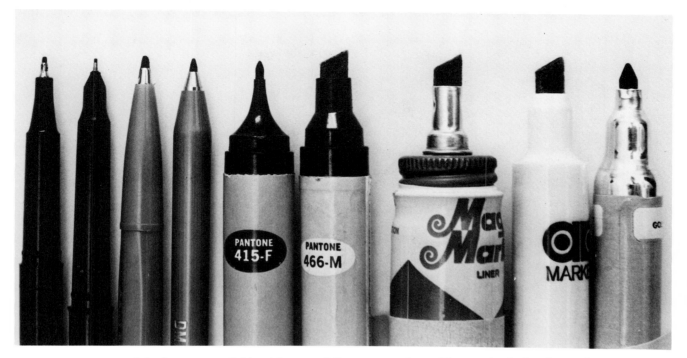

Markers are available with many different types of tips. The standard felt nib is multi-faceted and wedge-shaped. Other nibs are fine-pointed and are made from nylon or other plastic materials.

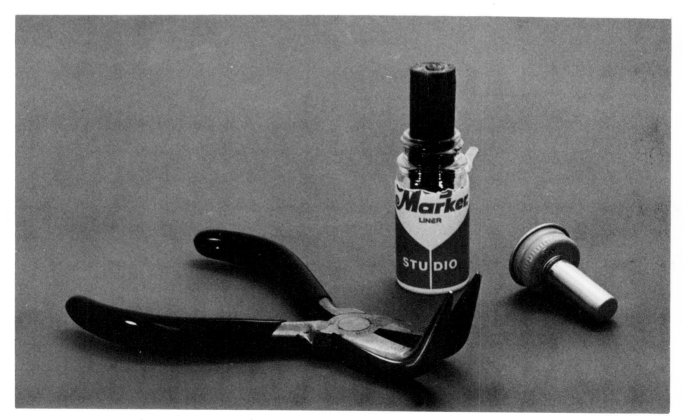

The Magic Marker Studio brand has the advantage of a removable cap and inner core, which can be used for painting large color areas by holding the core with a needle-nosed pliers.

MARKERS ON AQUABEE PLATE-FINISH BRISTOL

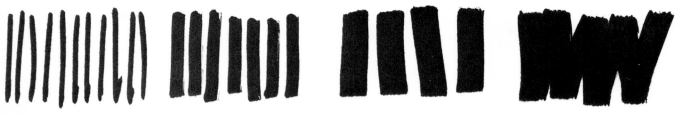

The nib on the Magic Marker is multifaceted, enabling you to create various line weights by using the nib at different angles.

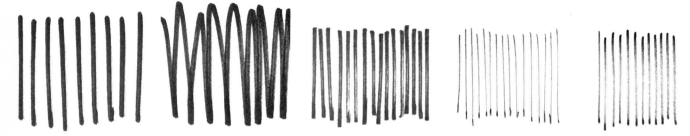

The first two examples (starting from the left) were done with a Markette Thinrite Marker. This nib is bullet-shaped and draws a fairly thin, even line. The rest of the lines were drawn with the Pantone fine-line marker, the Pilot Fineline, and the Pentel Sign Pen, in that order.

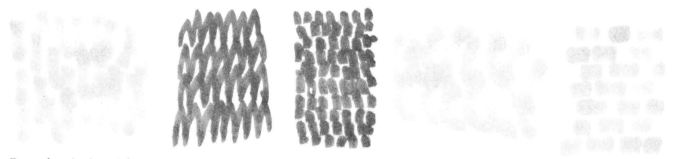

Examples of a few of the many marks and textures that can be produced with the Magic Marker nib.

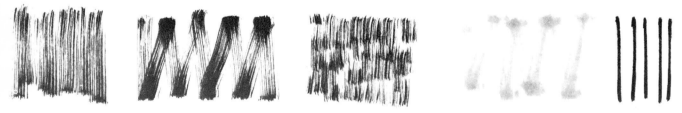

Marks produced by using a very dry marker. Don't discard old, dry markers—some interesting textures can be achieved with them.

MARKERS ON SYNTHETIC PAPER

How a gray Magic Marker handles on this paper.

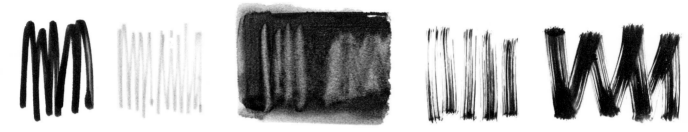

The first group of lines on the left was drawn with the Markette Thinrite. The next group was drawn with the Pantone fine-line pen, and the third example is a gray tone that has been cut back into with a lighter marker. Cutting back in like this works best on a paper where the markers do not soak in and the dyes are mostly on the paper surface. The last two examples in this line were done using a dry marker.

MARKERS ON RICE PAPER

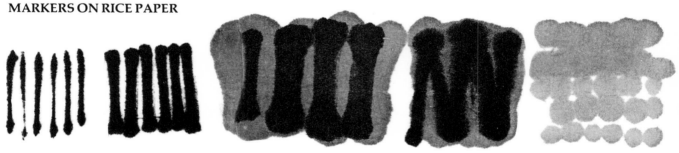

Marker dyes spread very rapidly on rice paper because of its absorbency. The first group of lines on the left were drawn very rapidly and remained thin. I drew the next group a little slower and the dyes spread, causing a fatter line. In the third group, I used a black over a gray that had dried thoroughly. The fourth group shows what happens when black is used over a tone that has not completely dried. The last example consists of dotting the paper with a marker nib. At the top of this group, I left the nib on the paper longer causing the dots to spread together. The lower dots were done very quickly and came out smaller.

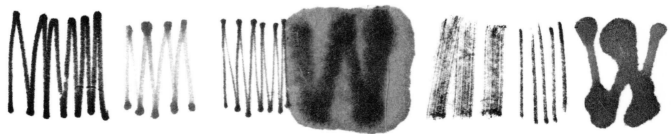

The first group on the left was done with a Markette Thinrite pen, the second with a Magic Marker Fineline pen, and the third with a Pantone fine-line pen. Next is a Magic Marker dark gray over a very wet lighter gray, resulting in more blending. The next two examples were drawn with a very dry marker. This type of line won't spread at all unless done on a very wet surface. In the last example, the dots on the ends of the lines occurred when I hesitated while drawing.

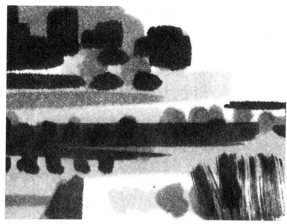

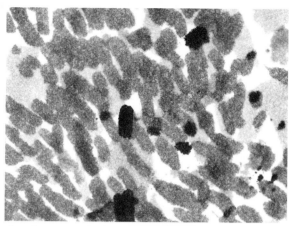

Various marks done over a gray tone on a high-quality layout paper. Markers go on this paper with a slightly softened effect, as the edges blend a bit.

Another example done on layout paper—the tones drawn on the white paper portion don't blend as much as those drawn over an existing tone.

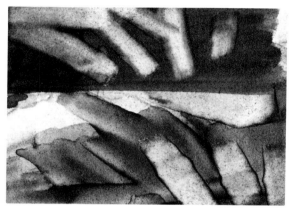

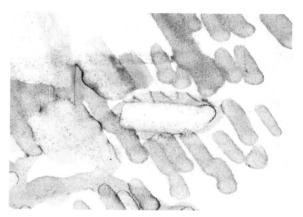

Tracing paper has a harder surface and is not as absorbent as layout paper. This enables you to rework darker areas by cutting back into them with lighter markers, as I have done here.

Markers used over a gray tone on tracing paper— there is no softening effect as on layout paper.

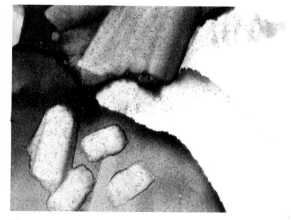

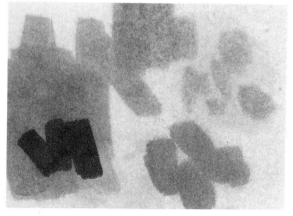

Tracing paper used with markers and solvent. In the dark area I have cut back in with a No. 1 gray.

Aquabee plate-finish Bristol has an excellent surface for markers. Here I demonstrate the soft effects achieved through using markers over one another.

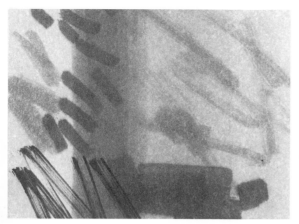

Another example done on Aquabee Bristol. Here I used a dry black and gray marker over blended tones.

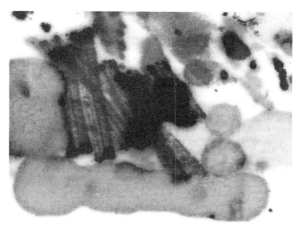

Markers on rice paper create an unusual effect that is impossible to achieve on other papers.

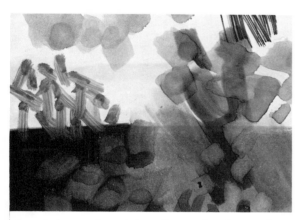

A coated paper is an interesting surface for marker painting. This surface is not quite as absorbent as others, allowing areas to be reworked easily.

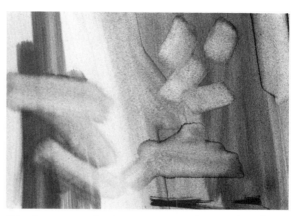

Kimdura, a synthetic paper, is another surface that allows tones and colors to be reworked.

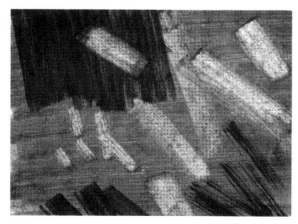

Canvasette is an interesting surface that simulates the surface texture of canvas. Frequently, the small recesses on the surface will hold more color, creating an interesting texture in the tones.

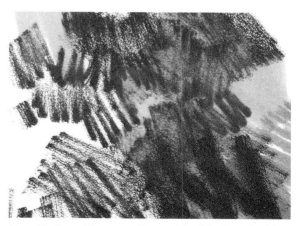

Coquille board is normally used for black and white ink and lithograph crayon drawings, but the markers take to this surface very well. When using a dry marker, take advantage of this unusual texture.

either dilute them with solvent or use them directly out of the can. I frequently use these inks or dyes with a brush.

Niji Giant Markers. Niji Giant Markers contain permanent ink and dry quickly. The extra-large ½" felt chisel tips are very handy for quick coverage of large areas. They are available individually or in a 12-color set.

Pantone Color Markers. Pantone Color Markers by Letraset come in 96 different colors that match the Pantone Color Matching System. Briefly, this system is used in the graphic arts and consists basically of matching printing inks, color tint overlays, color papers, and markers, each identified by a color number. For example, a graphic artist can design a brochure with a certain Pantone marker color and then be sure that in the final printing the colors will be correct because of the numbered color system.

Pantone Color Markers can be bought individually or in 12-color sets. The Pantone Art Director's set contains an assortment of 96 different colors and includes a stand.

Strathmark. This is a color marker line from Strathmore, the makers of fine papers. Their range of colors is quite extensive—200 are available. This marker has been designed to fit the hand naturally and is very comfortable. There is a large color label on the marker for easy color identification.

Steig Lightfast Watercolor Markers. This product is available in 20 water-based, oderless colors. These markers will be of special interest to artists who enjoy markers as a painting medium, as they are light-fast. This means that they will retain their quality without fading (indefinitely under certain ideal conditions). They are available in two sets of ten colors.

PAPERS

There are many papers that can be used to paint on with markers, since markers are compatible with most surfaces. I will recommend some personal choices, but they are by no means the only possibilities. You should experiment with many other papers—perhaps other surfaces will suit you better.

Layout Paper. I recommend that you use a very high-quality layout paper—don't use the cheaper brands. In my area, Detroit, Lewis Artist Supply has a very excellent pad available—the Lewis layout pad 864—which consists of very fine paper that takes markers very well. Another pad I like is the Beinfang Admaster. Both pads are available in various sizes, 100 sheets of paper to each pad.

Bristol Board. There are many fine Bristol boards made by Bainbridge, Aquabee, Strathmore, and Crescent. The Aquabee plate-finish Bristol has a very smooth surface that takes markers nicely. It's available in convenient pads of different sizes.

When using most Bristol boards with markers, be sure to use a backing sheet—the markers tend to bleed through.

Japanese Rice Papers. Rice papers work very well with markers. I especially like to use them because the marker colors saturate the paper surface which then stays wet longer, enabling the colors to be blended. The effects achieved on this surface are very much like that of a fresh watercolor.

Synthetic Paper. Many new synthetic, plastic papers are used in the printing industry. One of them is Kimdura, a very durable "paper," the surface of which is highly compatible with markers. While this paper is not sold in artist supply stores yet, you may be able to purchase it from a printing paper company. Hopefully, it will eventually be available for artists.

Crescent Acrylic Illustration Board. This board has a linenlike surface texture that takes markers nicely. This surface is normally used for painting with acrylic paint or designer's colors.

Other papers. Tracing papers are very fine for working with markers. The colors do not soak in as much as on other surfaces and can be reworked for some unusual effects Some watercolor papers can also be used with this medium—but stay away from the rough surfaces.

Generally speaking, markers work quite well on most surfaces, so experiment with the different boards and papers your local artist supply store stocks.

CHAPTER TWO

Basic Marker Techniques

THERE ARE MANY techniques that can be used to do marker paintings, and the examples in this chapter show some of the methods of working that I have experimented with. Markers can be used exclusively or can be effectively combined with graphite, charcoal, or china marking pencils, as well as with pen or brush for various effects. Often an outline drawing or outline accents are necessary for a successful marker rendition. In general, it is sometimes difficult to define objects through tone, as markers tend to have a soft look—strong shadows or contrasts in a scene can help alleviate this effect. Also, an overall effect that appears undefined can be clarified with the use of linear accents.

MIXING YOUR OWN COLORS

In addition to the regular markers, Flo-master inks and solvent can be used to mix your own colors. These inks, when used with a brush, produce an effect similar to watercolor. For the beginner, however, mixing colors and all the clean up involved can take all the fun and convenience out of marker painting. It's a good idea to wait until you develop and become more confident before you experiment with mixing marker inks and solvent. *A reminder:* when using solvents, you must have proper ventilation or work outside—the fumes can be stifling and dangerous.

CHOOSING A PAPER

Markers handle much differently than paint, and some paper surfaces simply do not take markers well. It's most important to use a paper surface that is compatible to the medium—the results can be pretty discouraging when attempting to paint on the wrong kind of surface.

For the examples in this chapter, I limited my choice of paper to five distinctly different surfaces: a high-quality layout paper, Japanese rice paper, high-surface Bristol board, coated paper, and a new plastic surface, a synthetic paper called Kimdura. (Please note that there are other plastic-surfaced papers besides Kimdura available.) All these five papers have excellent surfaces for doing marker paintings and each one yields effects that differ greatly from the others. Of course, there are many other papers and boards that can be used, and you should experiment with as many surfaces as possible.

SKETCHING

In the beginning, you may prefer doing rough sketches on-the-spot, making color notes, and then finishing your paintings at home. Or you might want to try doing very rough, on-the-spot sketches and taking color or black and white Polaroid photographs to use as reference for your finished paintings. At first, confine your efforts to fast, simple color sketches, and gradually work up to the point where you will be able to tackle a painting. This will take a certain amount of time, but the more you practice using markers, the sooner you will learn to master this medium.

Incidently, learning to properly use markers has a definite commercial value as well. Many advertising agencies and art studios use marker renderings for both preliminary layout work and television storyboards. If you are proficient in the medium, you might possibly turn this talent into a career.

USING THE MARKERS

Most of the following examples were done primarily using Magic Markers, as I have worked with this brand for years and am most familiar with their color range. On occasion, I have used AD markers and Pantone markers and have found them to be very good products with a vast range of available colors. With the Magic Marker brand, you can remove the inner fibrous material that contains the color (hold it with pliers so your finger won't become stained by the dye) and use it for brushing in very large flat tones. However, very large flat areas are almost impossible to render by using the marker nib itself. Try a couple of colors from each brand to make up your own mind as to which one suits you best. You can also mix them up, using different colors from the various makes.

At any rate, learning to use the markers is the important part, so study the following examples carefully. It would be good to duplicate the various effects, since these examples show how various subjects can be handled as well as demonstrate different marker painting techniques. The demonstrations in the following chapters show how to render a variety of subject matter graphically, step-by-step.

Pencil and tone. *This is probably the most basic marker technique and is a good one for you to start with. Draw a sketch with a pencil of medium grade, such as HB, and then fill in and build up the tones with markers. This particular example is rendered on Aquabee plate-finish Bristol, a very fine surface for pencil and markers. This sketch was done using only gray and black markers, as were most of the others in this chapter. When you first use markers, you should work mostly in black and white and attempt color later.*

Ink line and tone. *(Below) Here I combine ink line and markers—a technique that I also enjoy using with watercolors—on a plate-finish Bristol. The pen lines help to define the objects clearly, and the markers are used rather loosely over the whole picture, creating a nice effect. This is the technique I employ when doing marker renderings for advertising layouts and TV storyboards because it is a fast, clean way of presenting ideas. When doing advertising work, I invariably render on a high-quality layout paper with a technical pen for my basic drawing. Usually, these renderings must be rubber-cemented or otherwise mounted into a layout or book dummy, and a very thin paper insures a neater job.*

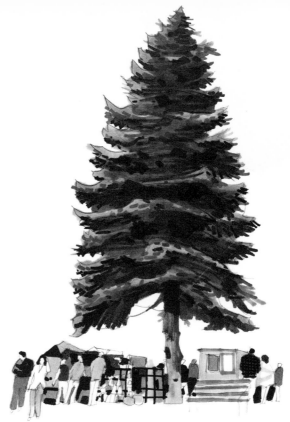

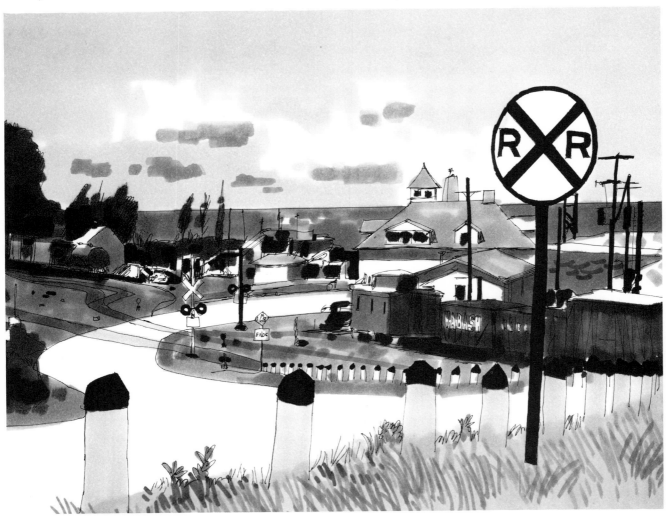

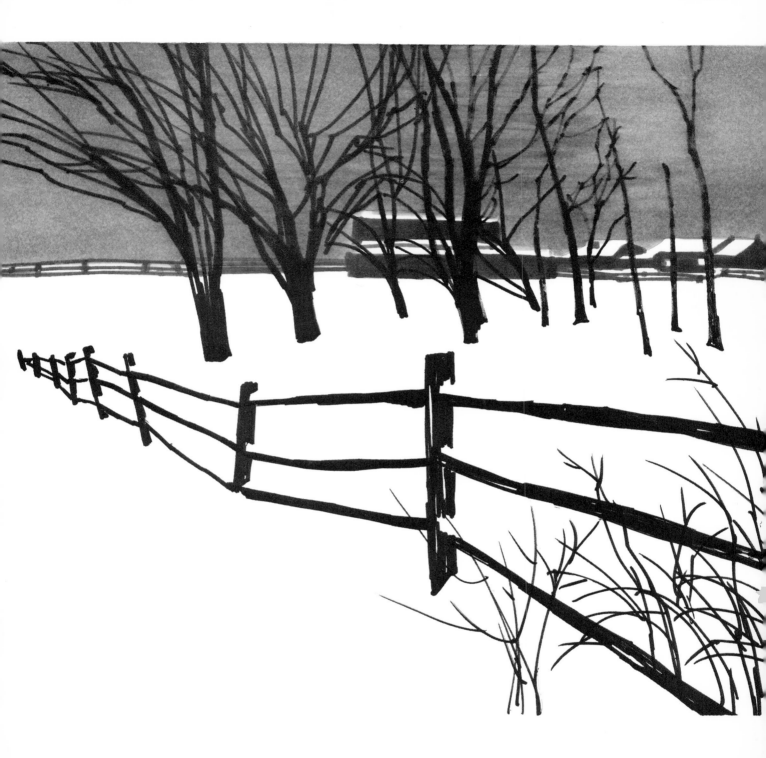

Marker line and tone. *Here is a snow scene done with only two shades of gray plus black. The fence and trees were drawn using a Design Art Marker, and the background buildings and fence were drawn with a No. 7 gray. The sky was put in last, using a No. 4 gray marker. It's rendered on Strathmore high-finish Bristol.*

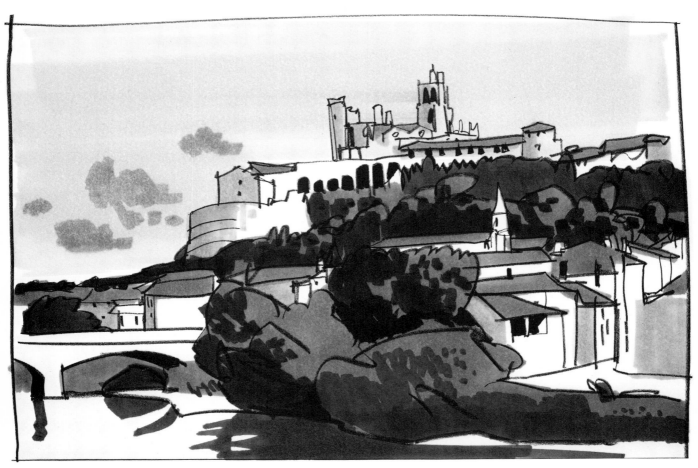

Charcoal pencil and tone.

(Above) Another medium that combines well with markers is the charcoal pencil, which works very nicely on a high or plate-finish Bristol. After you complete your charcoal drawing, spray it with workable fixative, so it won't smudge; then fill in the areas in which you want tone with markers. Another fast, effective marker technique.

Stabilo pencil and tone on coated paper. *There are many types of pencils and an even greater number of paper surfaces that can be used for marker paintings. This particular example was done on Lusterkote, a coated paper used for printing. It's a fine paper with a hard, glossy surface. My basic drawing was done using an All Stabilo pencil, which is similar to a lithograph or china marking pencil and can be used on most any surface. This is quite an interesting combination, as the markers tend to dissolve the pencil line.*

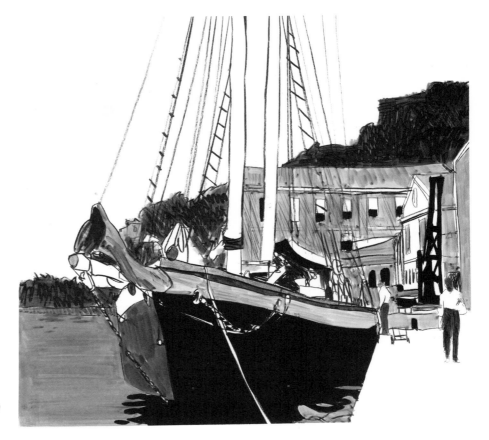

Tone and line accents on rice paper. *The black accents were put in first, using a black Pantone fine-line marker; then the grays were added. The sky was done by removing the fibrous materials inside the Magic Marker, holding it with pliers, and putting down very broad, bold strokes on the paper surface.*

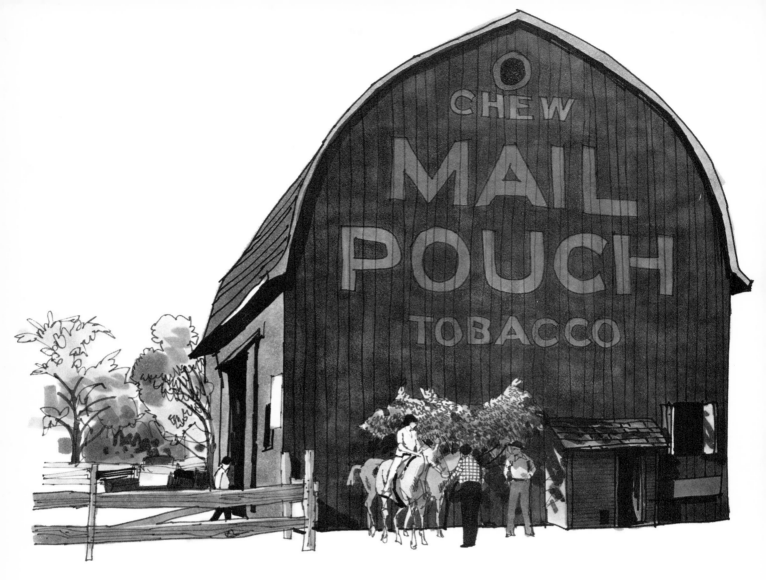

Fine line markers with tone. *(Above) This scene was drawn on a plate-finish Bristol board using a Pantone 417F gray fine-line marker for the figures, fence, and trees. For the barn, I used a black Pantone fine-line marker. After the basic drawing was complete, I carefully built up the gray values using Magic Marker grays. I used Nos. 2, 4, 5, and 7 grays as well as black for some accents. This example again illustrates how you can leave out certain parts of a picture, such as the sky and ground, and still have a painting that looks right.*

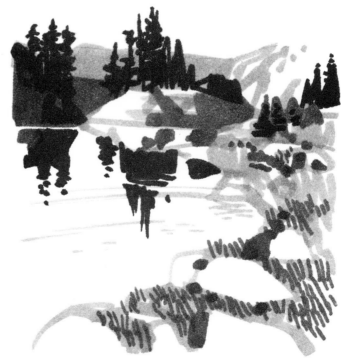

Tone on layout paper. *This sketch was done using Nos. 2, 5, 7, and 9 grays. The white areas are very important in this picture, and add a great deal of sparkle. The short strokes in the foreground simulate a textured grass area, and just a few simple strokes and tree reflections create a good illusion of water.*

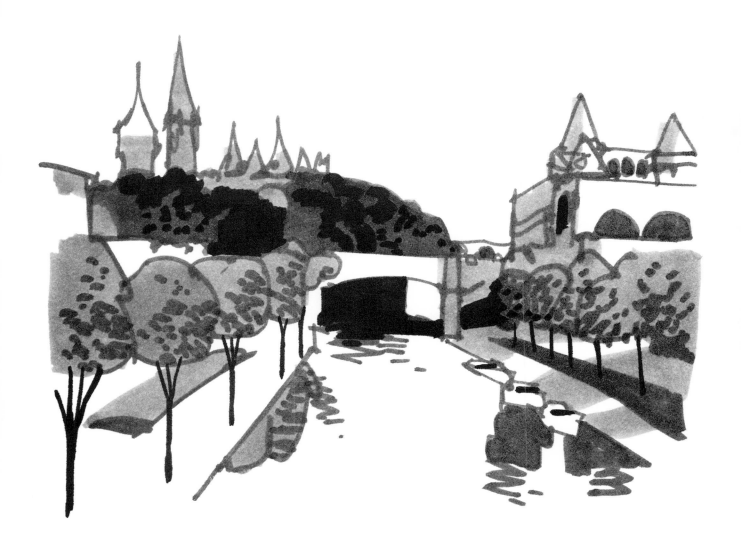

Tone line and tone on layout paper. *This scene was drawn with a No. 7 gray marker on a high-quality layout paper, a very fine surface for marker paintings. The other tones were added with grays Nos. 5 and 9.*

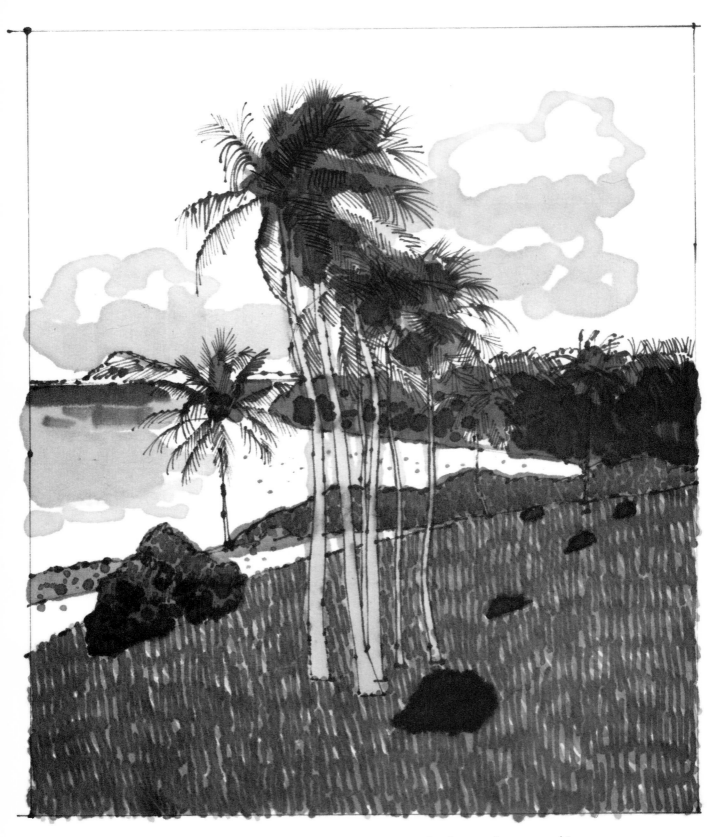

Fine line and tone on rice paper. *A Pantone 417F gray fine-line marker was used for the basic drawing here, and the paper is rice paper. The tones were put in using Magic Marker grays Nos. 2,3,5,7, and 9. The cloud effects were achieved by drawing slowly on the paper surface so the tones would spread freely.*

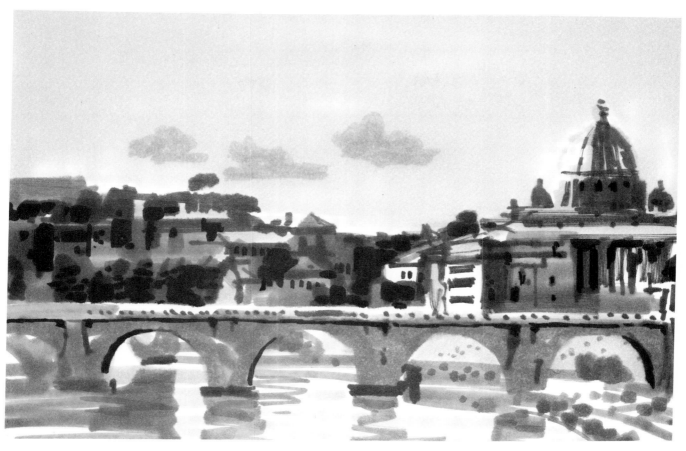

Tone on Bristol board. (Above) Again, in this scene I used grays Nos. 2,5,7, and 9. The smooth sky, done by using the fibrous material from inside the marker bottle. This is done with a broad stroke by holding the core with pliers.

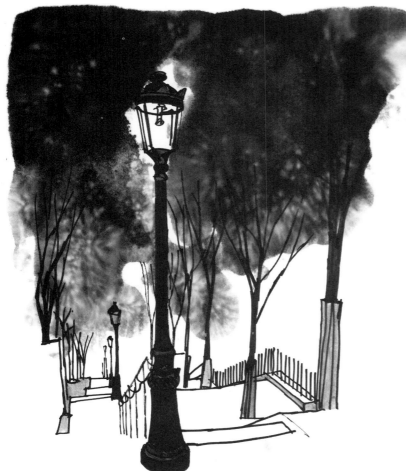

Marker line and tone with solvent.
This example is done on a coated paper using Flo-master black ink and solvent. I diluted the black ink with solvent and washed it onto the paper with a large watercolor brush. While this was still wet, I dripped on first more ink and then some solvent. After it dried, I was not satisfied with the result until I turned the paper over—the marker ink had bled through, creating just the interesting wet effect I was after. Then I finished the painting on this reverse side of the paper.

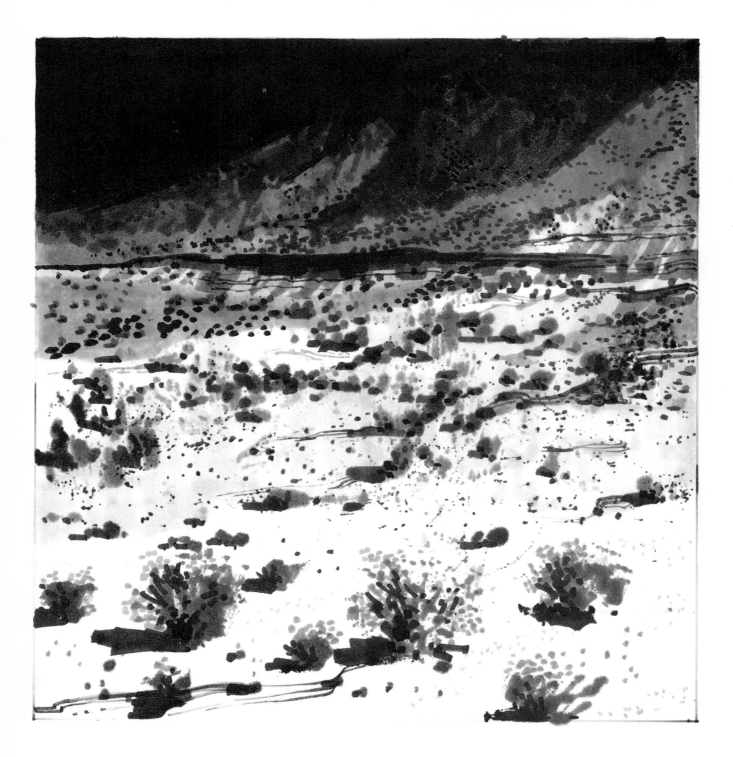

Tone and accidental effects. *For the two of the marker paintings done on rice paper, I used a backing sheet of high-finish Bristol. Some very interesting textures and effects resulted from the markers bleeding through. In this particular case, the effect reminded me of a southwestern desert scene. Working directly on the backing sheet—adding a few shadows here and there and a mountain in the background—the scene developed quickly. Keep an open mind, and you will be able to incorporate many of these unusual effects, found on the backing sheets, in your work.*

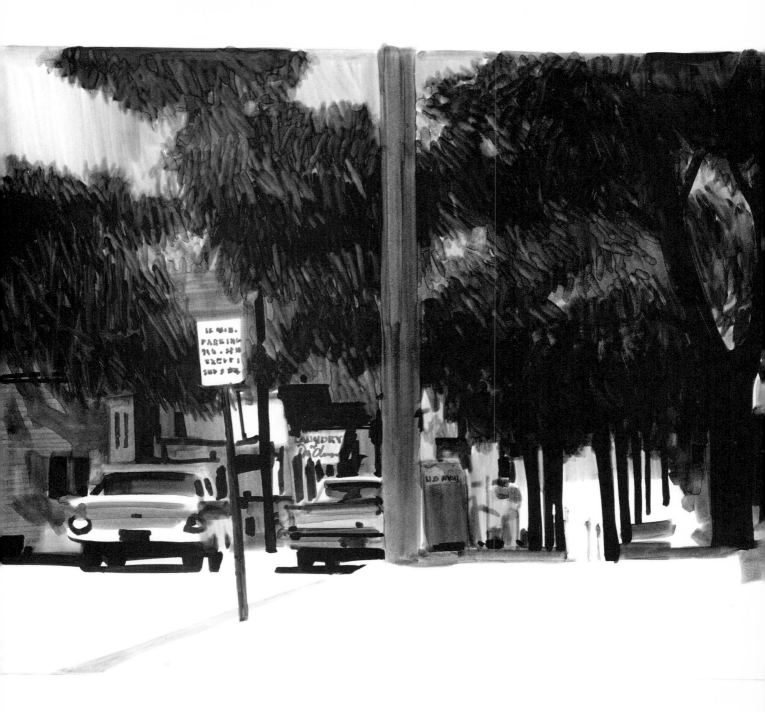

Tone on synthetic paper. *Kimdura is a plastic paper (one of many) used in the printing industry and is an excellent surface to use for marker paintings. I started by rendering
the very dark areas with a No. 9 gray. Then with a No. 2 gray, I stroked back into the
darks, creating a leaflike texture. On this surface, the markers do not soak in as much,
and it's easy to cut back into dark tones with lighter grays or colors.*

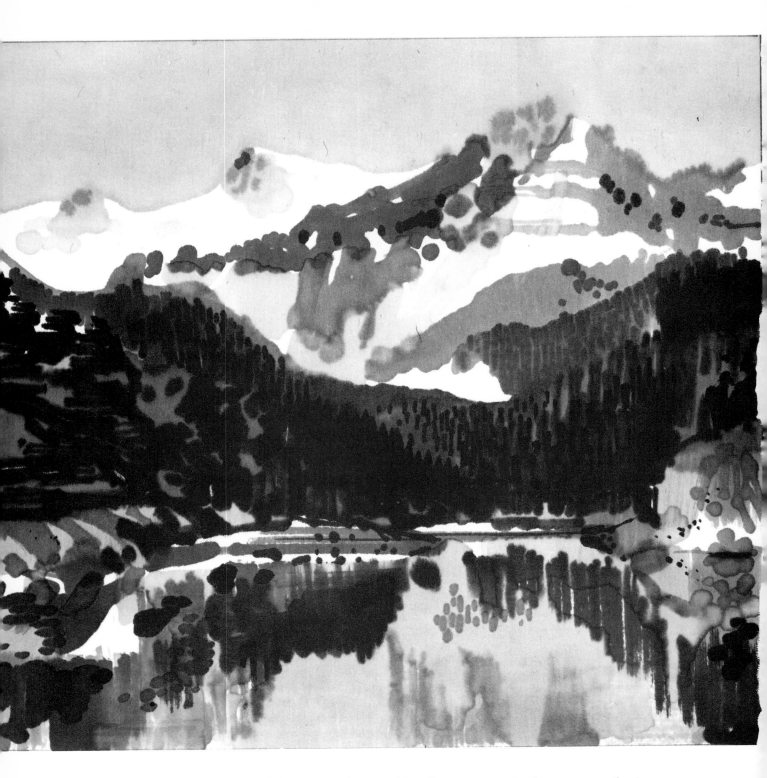

Tone on rice paper. (*Above*) *I started this painting by putting in washes of dark gray with a No. 7 Magic Marker. Then I added the sky and other intermediate tones, being very careful to leave a few white areas for contrast. Last, I put in the very dark parts and tree textures. The softness that can be achieved on rice paper is virtually impossible to duplicate on other surfaces.*

Fine line, tone, and solvent on synthetic paper. (*Right*) *This study was first drawn with a black Pantone fine-line marker. The dark and light tones were put in with Magic Marker grays, solvent being used over the tones to soften the effect. The darker accents were added last with a black and a No. 9 marker.*

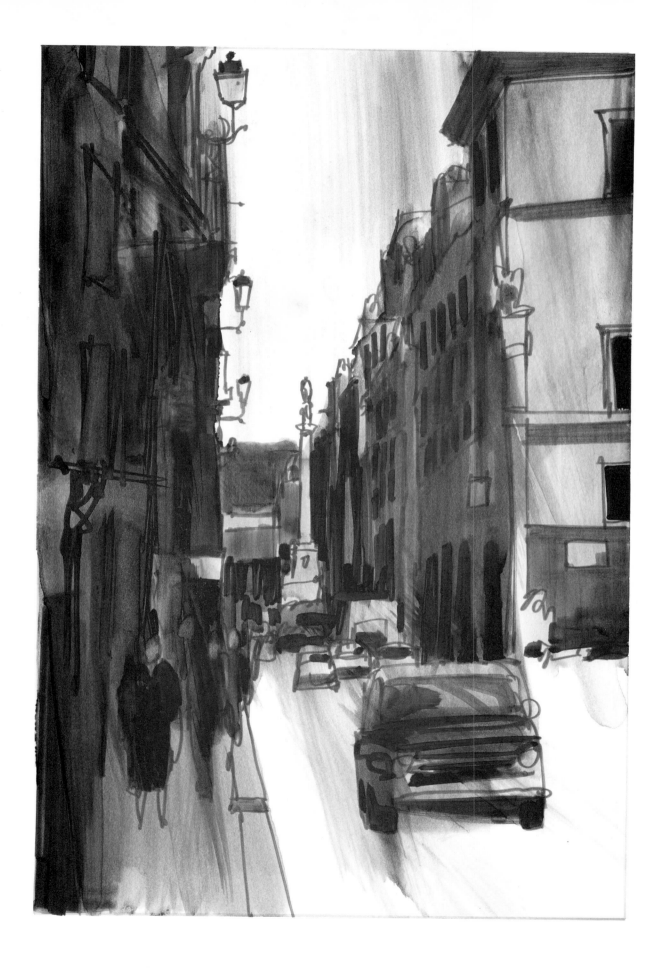

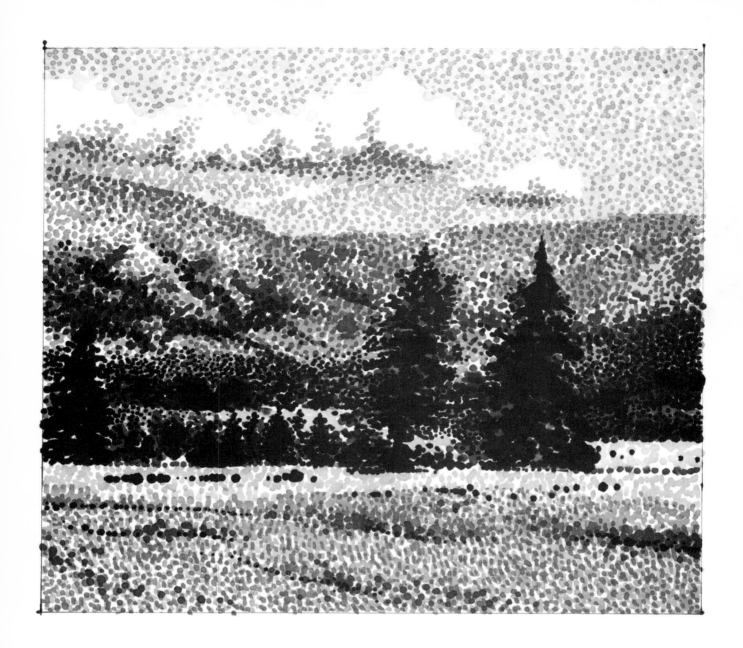

Pointillism on rice paper. *The pointillist technique is perfect for painting on rice paper, as the marker ink tends to spread in a perfect dot shape. Of course, the longer you leave the point touching the paper, the larger dot spreads. This effect can lead to some unusual patterns—experiment with various dot sizes on the same painting as a variation of this technique. Before starting a painting of this type, do a small value sketch to use as a guide for building up the various tones. This preliminary guide can be done using either pencil tones or markers.*

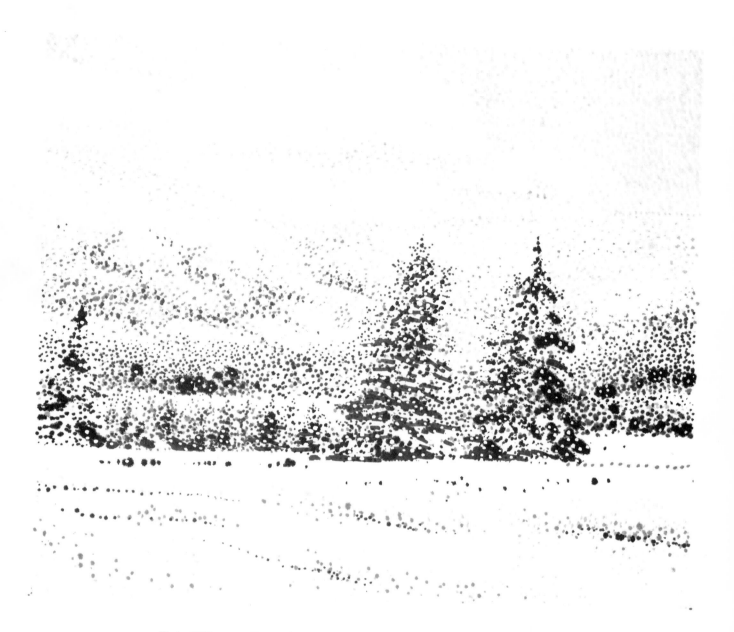

Pointillism on Bristol. *This painting is actually the backing sheet that I used while doing the previous painting. After I added the sky and a few dots of white paint on the dark shadows, I had a perfect winter version of the summer scene. Another example of how you can incorporate accidental effects in paintings.*

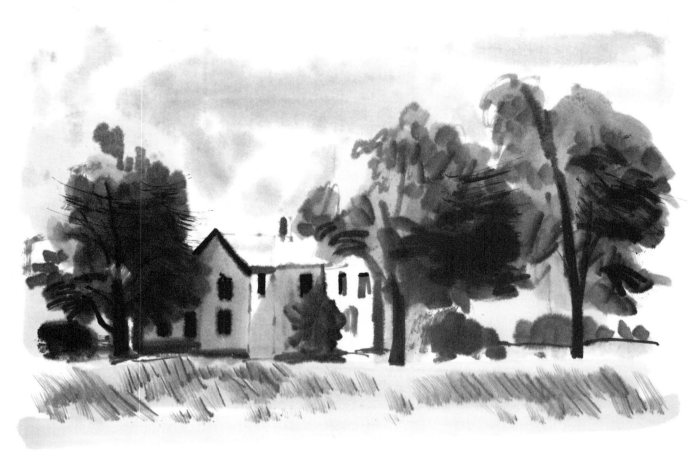

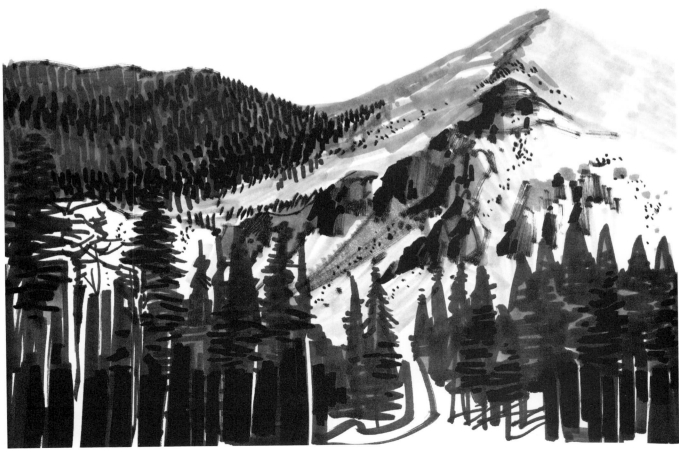

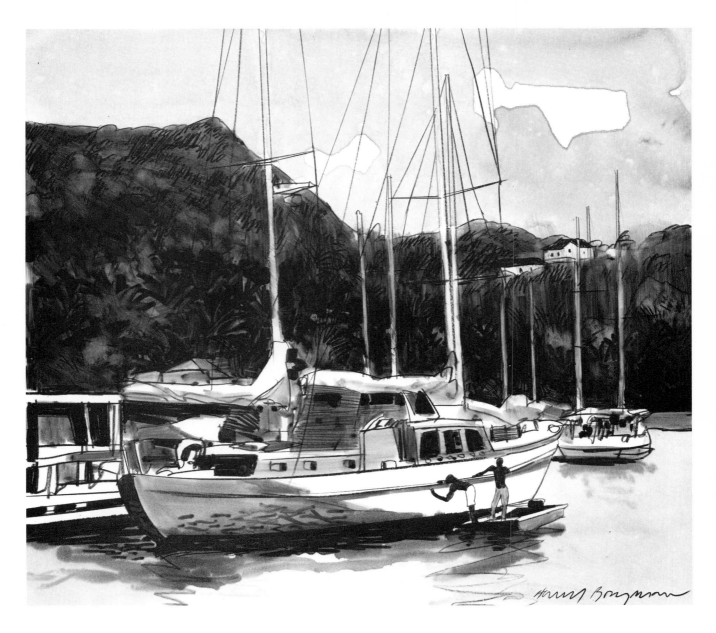

Tone and solvent on Bristol board. *(Above left) I used a brush and diluted Flo-master black ink for this quick sketch, mixing the tones on a tray. While this sketch is quite loose, more detailed work can also be done using this method—if you can stand the odor of the solvent! It's very strong, and you must be sure to have proper ventilation. Flo-master inks are available in several basic colors, which can be mixed to create your own hues and tones. It is much more trouble than painting with conventional markers, because you must clean your brushes and mixing tray.*

Bold stroke technique. *(Left) With this technique, you make the most out of the natural bold strokes that can be done with the marker nib. Certain subjects, such as trees, rocks, and grasses, lend themselves well to this method of working. Don't attempt to blend tones, but rather use the strokes themselves as part of the overall design.*

Combining techniques. *(Above) Here is an example that successfully combines some of the different techniques shown in Chapter 2. I did the basic drawing with a Stabilo pencil on a synthetic paper. The sky and water were put in with a brush using diluted Flo-master ink. The background tones were added with Nos. 7 and 9 Magic Marker grays, after which I cut back into the dark tones with a No. 5 gray. The effect yielded the look of palm trees. I also brushed some drops of solvent onto the background—when dry, they gave the impression of another type of foliage. I finished off the background by adding a little texture to the hills with the pencil. The intermediate tones were then put into the foreground dock and ships, finishing the painting.*

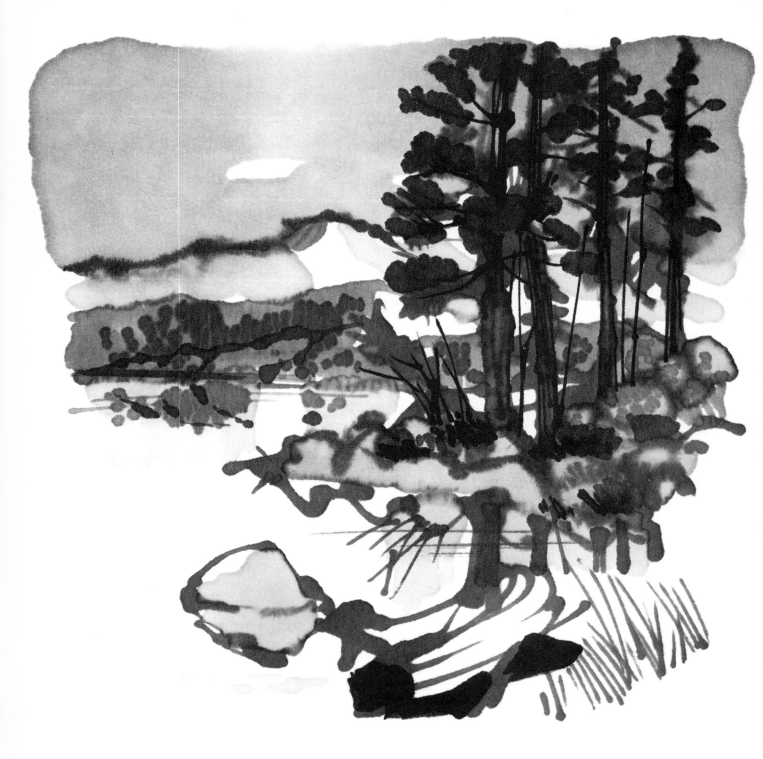

Tone line and tone on rice paper. *An unusual surface that can be used for marker paintings is Japanese rice paper, which I first used for printing woodcuts and now find to be excellent surfaces for marker paintings. On rice paper, the markers tend to spread and stay wet longer, creating softer effects generally. This quick sketch is not unlike a watercolor in character. When working on this paper, always use a backing sheet of heavier paper or board, as the markers bleed through the rice paper.*

CHAPTER THREE

Painting Trees with Markers

MANY TECHNIQUES are suitable for painting trees with markers. You can work in masses, using a very bold style, or you can do highly detailed work, delineating every leaf. In this chapter, there are several examples of tree renderings for you to examine. One technique that especially lends itself to painting trees is the pointillist technique, shown in Demonstration 2. The carefully placed dots used in this style create a realistic leaflike texture. Other techniques covered are line and tone, bold stroke, underpainting, and some examples of very loosely rendered trees.

In the beginning, you may feel that trees are very difficult to paint. Carefully study all the examples in this chapter, and practice by copying some of them. By actually duplicating these renderings, you will learn a great deal about how they were done. This type of practice will show you how simple some of these paintings are—they often consist of only three or four gray tones. From there you can go on to painting from photographs and even try some outdoor sketching.

When first beginning to paint trees, do them without any background until you feel confident enough to paint a complete scene. Perhaps you have a yard or live near a tree-filled park where you can sketch right on-the-spot. If you don't have ready access to trees, or if you don't feel at ease sketching outdoors, take a few Polaroid photographs to use as reference and draw indoors.

I would suggest starting your first paintings by making a light pencil sketch of the tree, in outline form. Then fill in the masses with gray markers as I have done in Demonstration 1. After you get acquainted with this method, try a few sketches without the pencil outline as I have done in *Birch tree* on page 47. Another thing that will help is to do close-up sketches of different trees, simulating the various bark textures.

The important thing, of course, is to keep practicing with your markers to gain confidence and learn what these tools can do. By the way, don't throw away any of your first attempts. It's interesting to compare your later efforts with them. If you practice, even a little bit, I know you will be surprised at the improvement in your work.

DEMONSTRATION 1. MAPLE TREE: PENCIL AND TONE

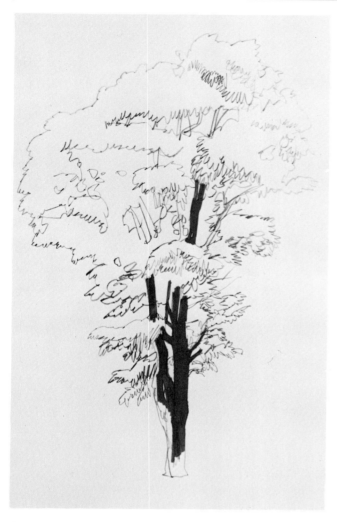

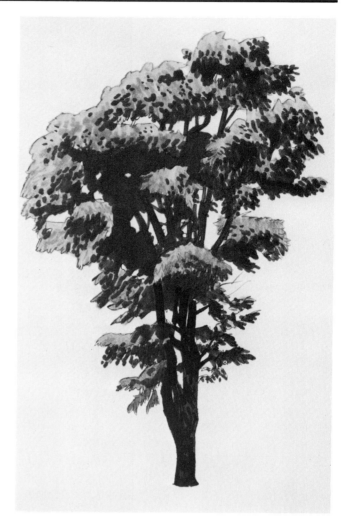

Step 1. *I start this painting by first doing a pencil drawing on plate-finish Bristol board. The drawing is simple, without any shading—this is the way you should approach your first attempts. Here I have started to put in the dark tones of the tree trunk.*

Step 2. *I use a No. 5 gray to put in an overall value on the leaves. Then I use a No. 7 gray to put in the shadow tones. This is quite easy, as I am simply filling in the outline drawing.*

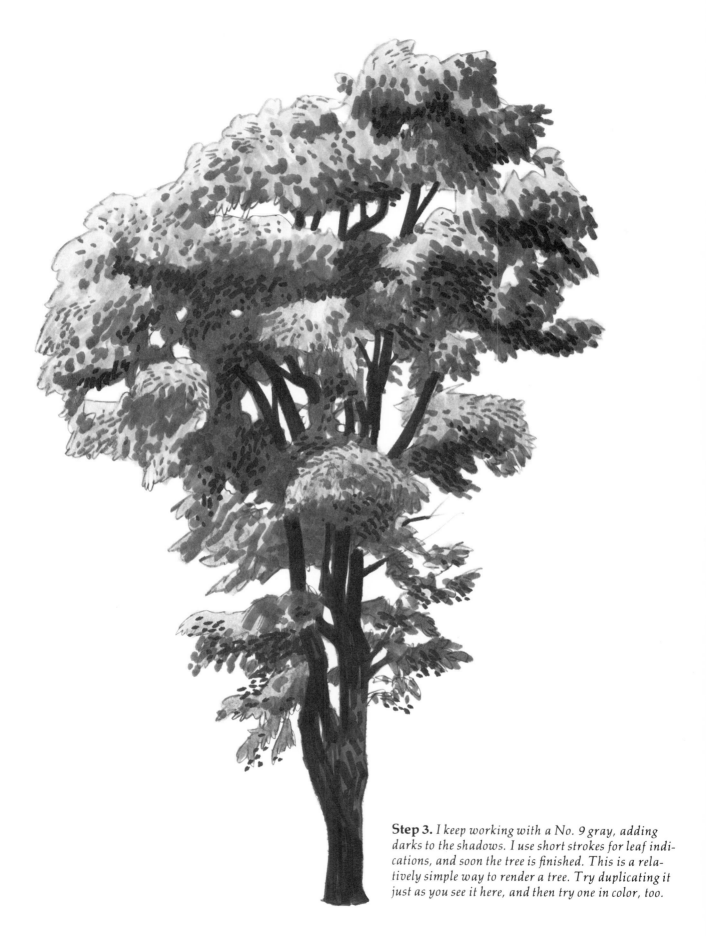

Step 3. *I keep working with a No. 9 gray, adding darks to the shadows. I use short strokes for leaf indications, and soon the tree is finished. This is a relatively simple way to render a tree. Try duplicating it just as you see it here, and then try one in color, too.*

DEMONSTRATION 2. COTTONWOOD TREE: POINTILLIST TECHNIQUE

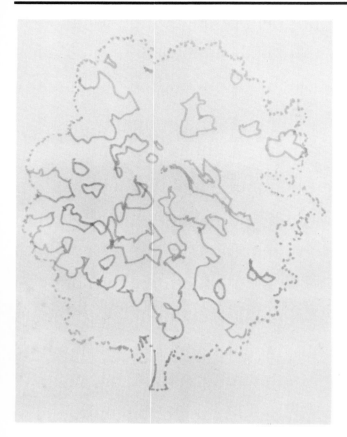

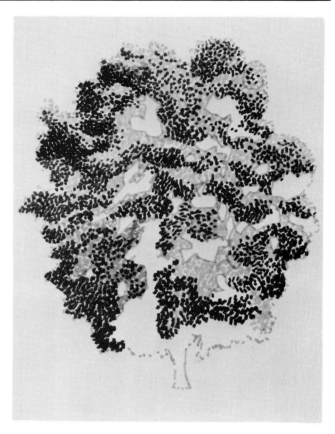

Step 1. *This is the best way to start a rendering in the pointillist style—simply do a dotted outline of the tree with a light gray marker. If I were working in color, a light green would have worked fine. Notice that I have indicated where the shadows fall on the leaves.*

Step 2. *I gradually work up the tones with Nos. 4, 5, and 7 grays. The tree is starting to look right. In the upper right section of leaves, I have started to add a darker shadow tone.*

Step 3. *(Right) I keep building up the darker tones, coming back with the intermediate grays where necessary, until the painting is finished. This is an interesting but time-consuming technique. You must remember to work very carefully, so all the dots end up relatively the same size. This technique works very well on most paper surfaces—try it on rice paper for an unusual effect.*

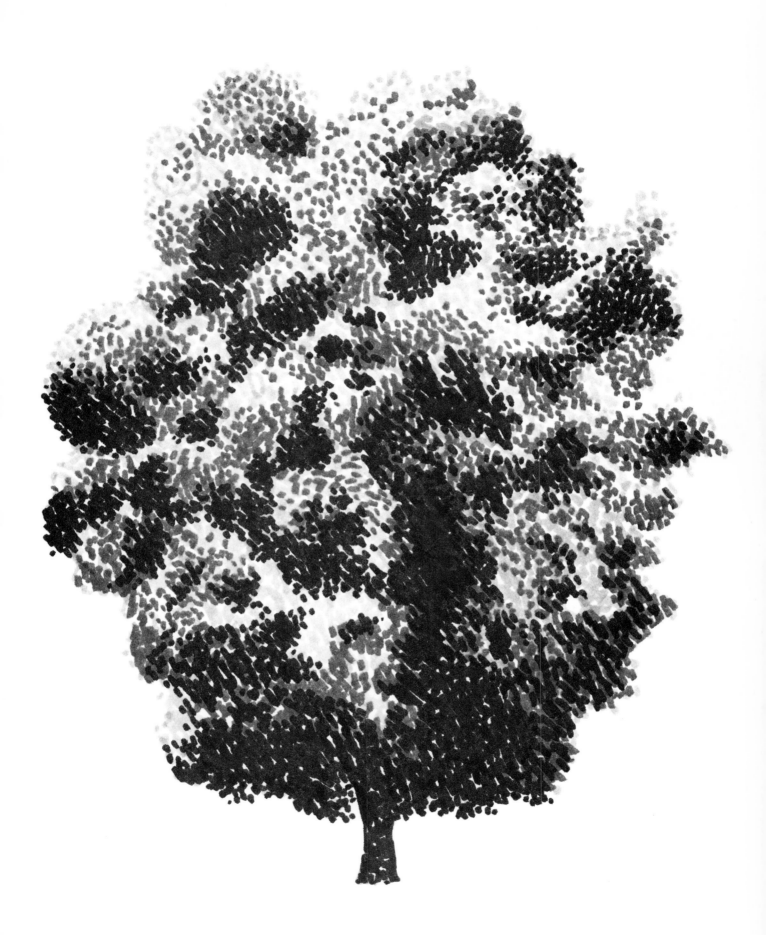

DEMONSTRATION 3. PINE TREES: CHINA MARKING PENCIL

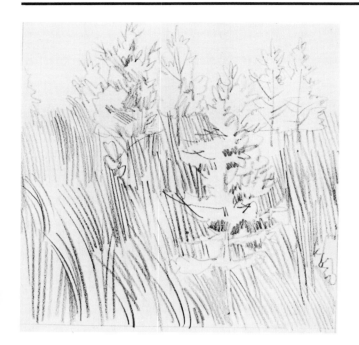

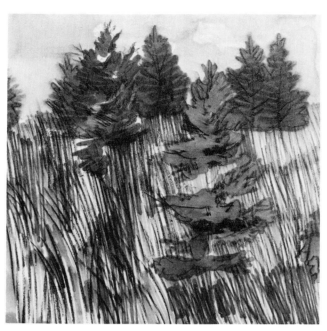

Step 1. *I begin by doing a fast, loose sketch on the rice paper with a china marking pencil. Litho crayon or an ALL Stabilo pencil would also work well. I have indicated some of the grass texture, but the trees are simple outlines with little detail.*

Step 2. *A No. 2 gray is used to put in the sky tone, and the grass texture is done by using a No. 5 marker with very bold strokes. The trees are filled in with a flat tone—while they are still a little wet, a darker tone is added. By working fast, the tones will blend nicely. A few darks in the grass area add a little depth.*

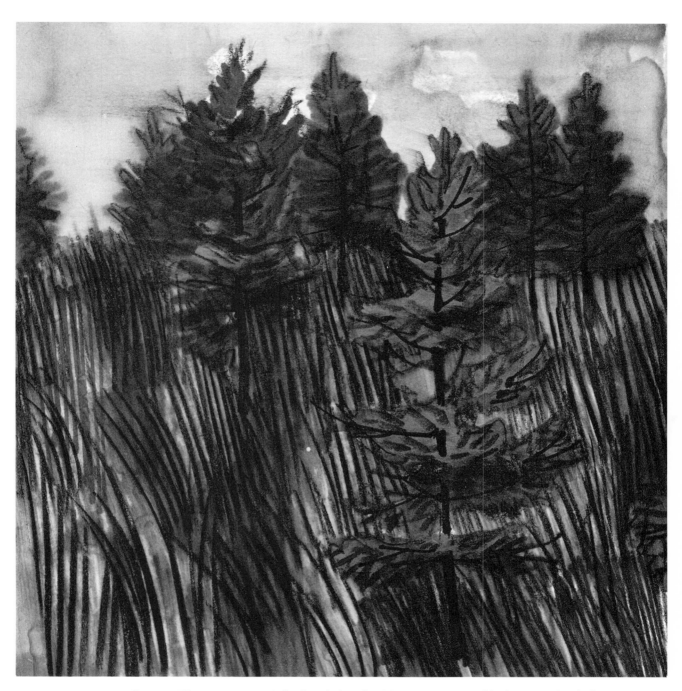

Step 3. *The trees are carefully detailed with a No. 9 gray. A few black accents finish the painting, which is done in a particularly loose style.*

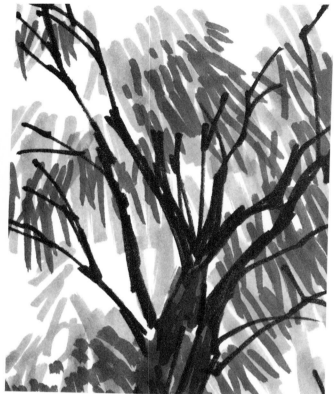

Willow tree: Bold stroke technique. *This is a very straightforward technique with no attempt to blend tones to hide strokes. Four markers were used for this sketch—grays Nos. 5, 7, and 9 and black—done on a sheet of plate-finish Bristol. A few simple black strokes on the tree trunks indicate a bark texture. The detail at left is reproduced the actual size it was rendered, so you can closely study the strokes used.*

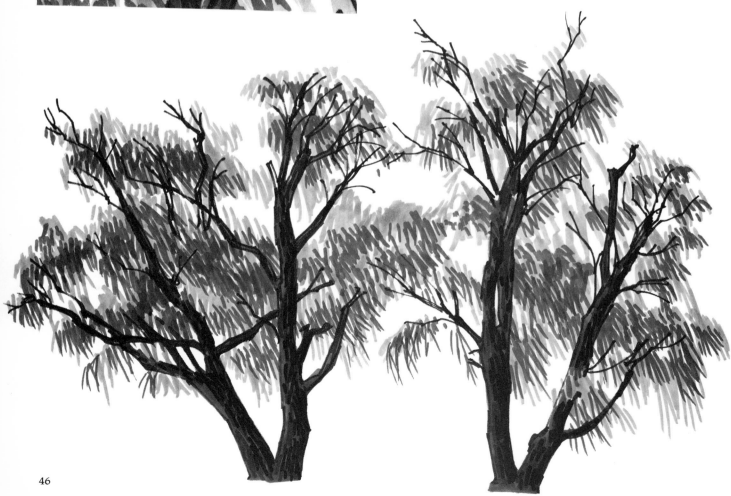

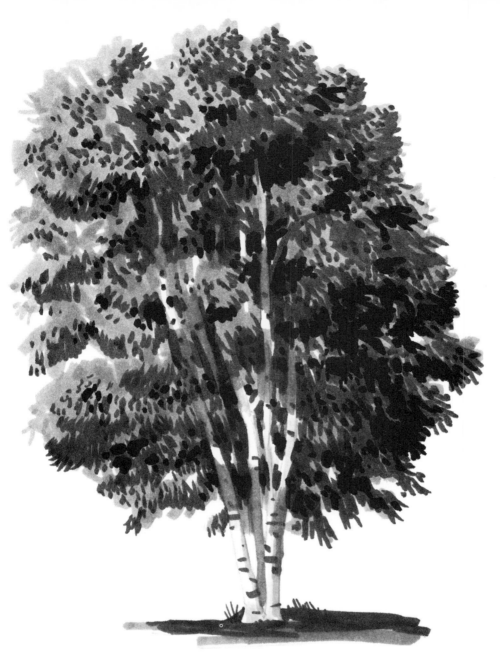

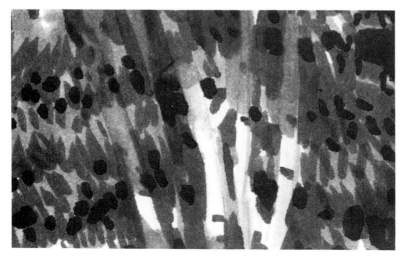

Birch tree: Tone on layout paper. *A tone rendering using Nos. 3, 5, and 7 grays and black. The basic shapes were done with the No. 3 gray—I was very careful to leave a few white areas for the tree trunk. When using markers, you must always plan to leave white paper surface showing through where you want a white tone. Here, I built up the darker tones gradually using short strokes in a zigzag motion for a leaf effect. A few shadows on the trunk finished the tree.*

In the actual size portion of the rendering, you can see how I have left the white paper showing through for the desired birch bark effect. A few little dark strokes add to the illusion of the bark texture.

Horsechestnut tree: Underpainting technique. *I used India ink and a brush to do the basic underpainting in this example. The ink brushstrokes were used to bring out the shadows and leaf textures. Then gray tones were added right over the ink rendering by first putting in an overall tone with a No. 4 gray marker and then adding the other tones carefully with Nos. 5, 7, and 9 grays. This technique works very well on many types of board surfaces. On the detail at right, you can see that I used a brush with split ends, which worked well for the strokes representing leaves.*

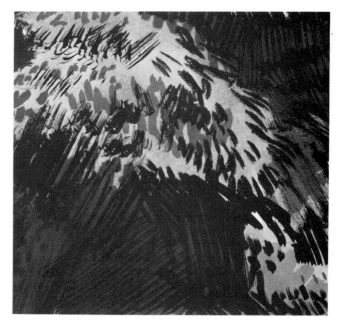

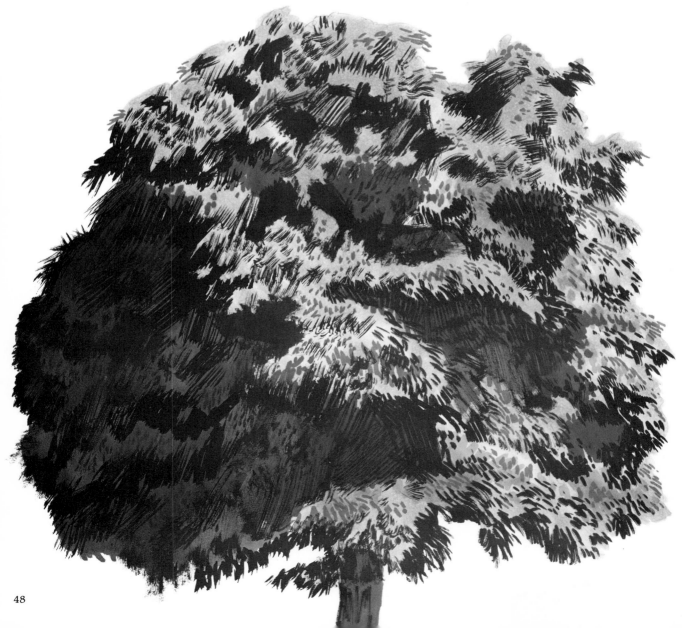

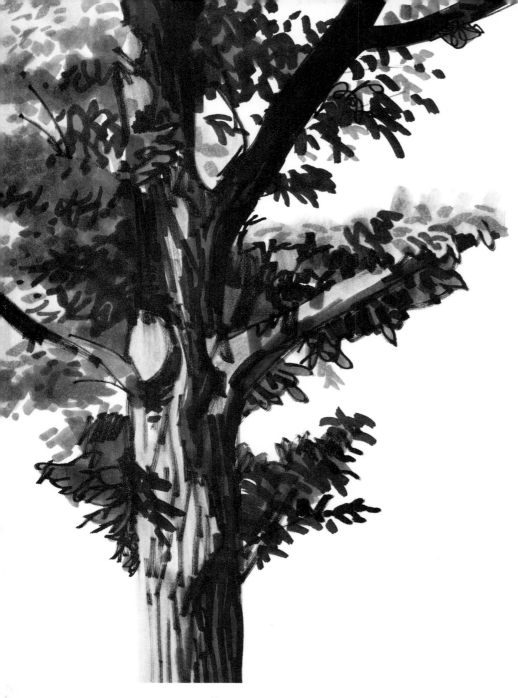

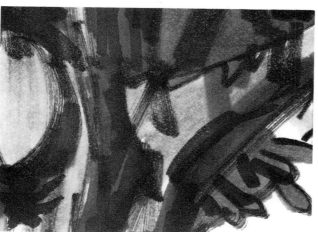

Close-up of white ash: Tone on Bristol board. *The basic drawing for this example was done with a Magic Marker that had a dry nib. This caused the lines to have a nice, soft drybrush effect, which worked very well for the bark texture. The leaves were put in with bold strokes, and the tones and shadows were added to the trunk with dark grays. The detail at left clearly shows the softness of the dry marker strokes.*

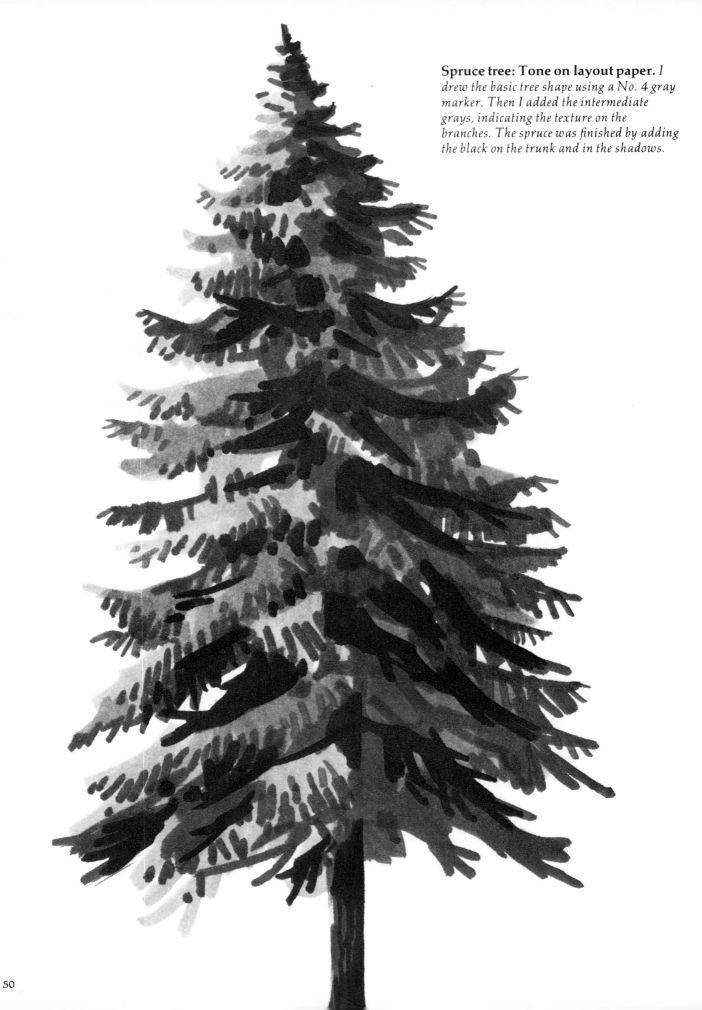

Spruce tree: Tone on layout paper. *I drew the basic tree shape using a No. 4 gray marker. Then I added the intermediate grays, indicating the texture on the branches. The spruce was finished by adding the black on the trunk and in the shadows.*

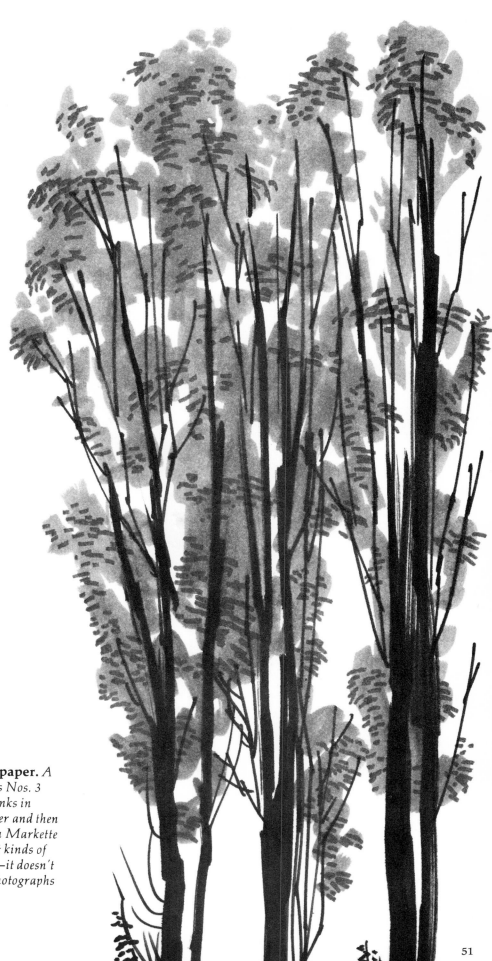

Poplar trees: Tone on layout paper. *A very quick sketch done using grays Nos. 3 and 7 and black. I put the tree trunks in boldly with a black Magic Marker and then added the thinner branches with a Markette pen. Practice doing many different kinds of trees using this sketchy technique—it doesn't matter if you are working from photographs or sketching on-the-spot.*

Flowers: Tone technique. *I started the flowers by painting in a background with a No. 7 gray, leaving the white flower shapes. Then I added the light gray shadows to the flowers and finished the background shadow detail with a No. 9 gray.*

CHAPTER FOUR

Grasses and Other Growing Things

WHEN PAINTING landscapes, you will be confronted with the necessity of rendering a great variety of grasses, flora, and undergrowth. Many subjects in this category, such as a field of corn or a mass of weeds, appear quite complex. When painting involves subjects such as these, think in terms of textural mass rather than individual plants. In other words, try to visualize your subject as a mass and interpret the surface characteristics with the markers.

This probably sounds easier said than done, but I will show you a few methods to use that are quite simple. For instance, short, thin strokes rendered over a tone can convey the impression of grass. You can experiment with all kinds of strokes over a tone that will look like bushes or masses of flowers. In fact, if you review the chapter on trees, you will see that the methods shown for rendering leaves can also be employed for these subjects. You can also study photographs of fields and bushes, patches of flowers, and other subjects. Analyze the different textures and try to duplicate them with your markers. This will help you understand just how the examples in this chapter were done.

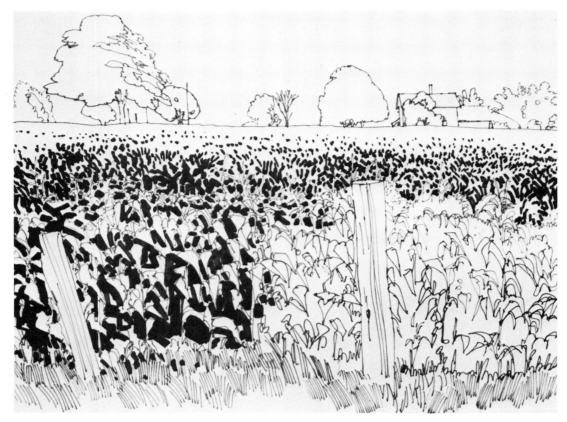

1

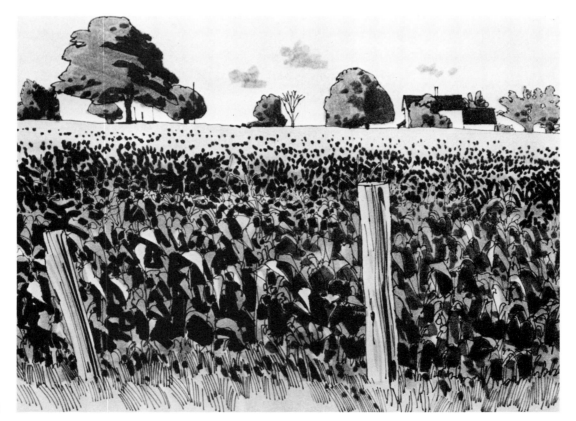

2

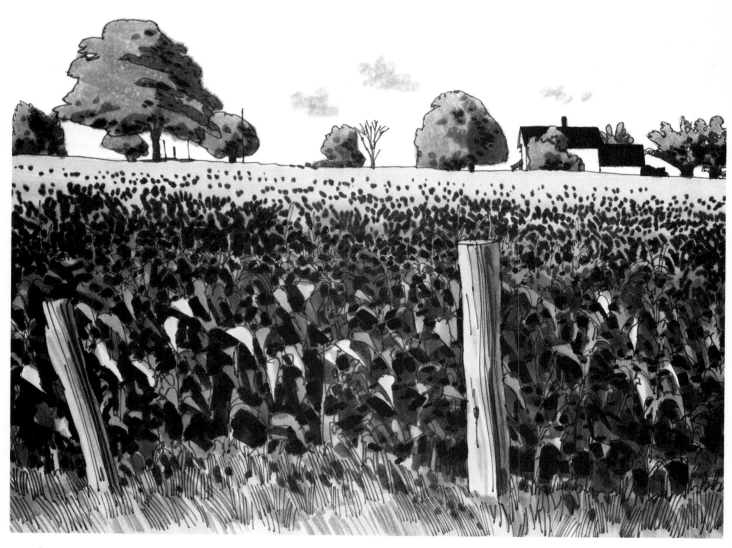

3

Step 1. *I did the basic drawing here carefully with a Pantone 417F fine-line pen. Then I put in the dark gray tones with a No. 7 gray Magic Marker. The grass texture in the foreground is also done with the Pantone pen.*

Step 2. *I add the background trees, sky, and clouds and put in shadow tones with the No. 7 gray. Next I put two tones of gray over the field area, the lighter tone in the distant part of the cornfield and the darker gray in the foreground. This contrast helps to create the illusion of depth.*

Step 3. *I sketched in darker shadow accents with a No. 9 gray throughout the whole field to complete the painting.*

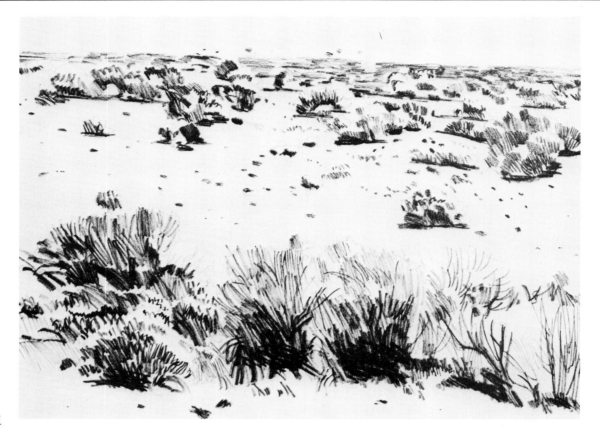

1

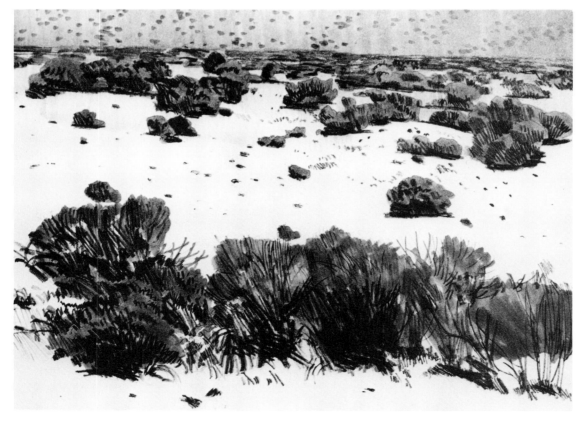

2

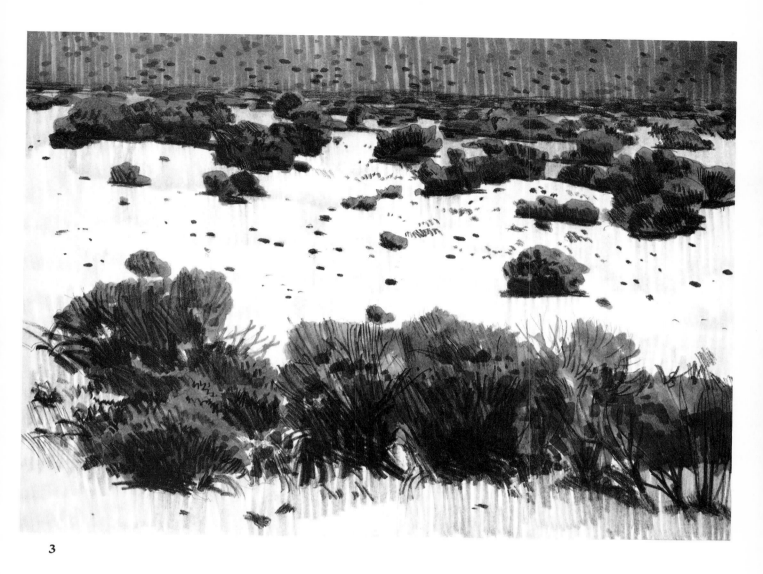

3

Step 1. *I use 4B charcoal pencil to do the underdrawing on a plate-finish Bristol board. This is a fine surface to use and is excellent for graphite pencils as well.*

Step 2. *A No. 5 gray is used to put a tone on the bushes, and a No. 7 on the darker shadow areas. Then I put a No. 3 gray tone on the distant slope and spotted a few bushes with a No. 5 gray marker. Next I start to add a light tone to the foreground area.*

Step 3. *The foreground tones are completed, and a few darker tones are added in the shadows for depth. In this rendering, I made no attempt to keep the tones smooth. This kind of an effect—when used throughout a painting—looks right and adds a little interest to the scene. Notice that the markers smudged some of the charcoal lines, creating an effect that is not objectionable.*

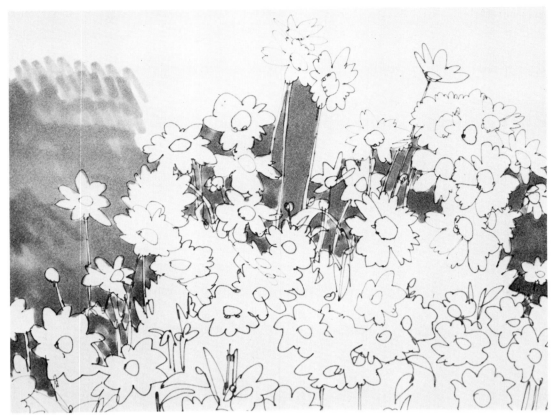

1

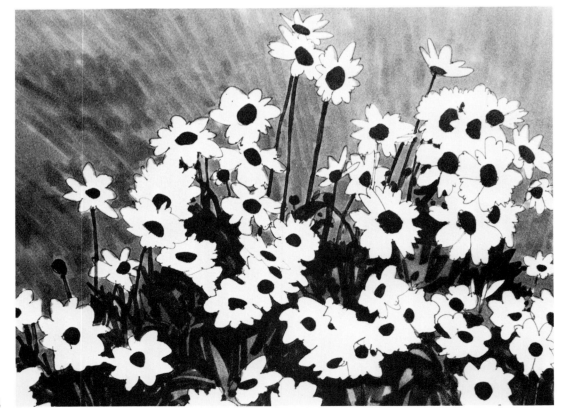

2

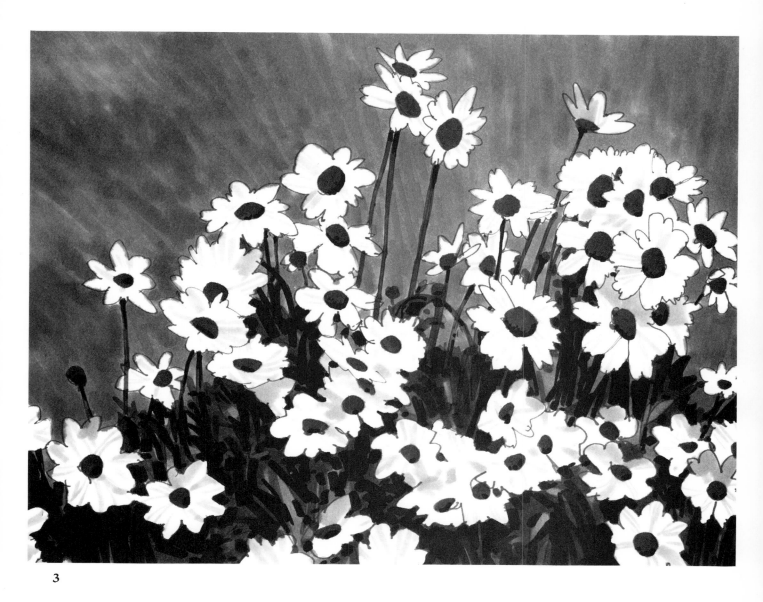

3

Step 1. *I start to put in a background tone with a No. 5 gray behind the outline drawing which is done with a Pantone 417F marker.*

Step 2. *After the background tone is completed. I use a No. 7 gray on the centers of the flowers and over the leaves.*

Step 3. *Here I put a light shadow tone on the flower petals, and I accent the shadow areas with a No. 9 gray. Then I go over the whole background again with a No. 5 gray to smooth out the uneven tone a little.*

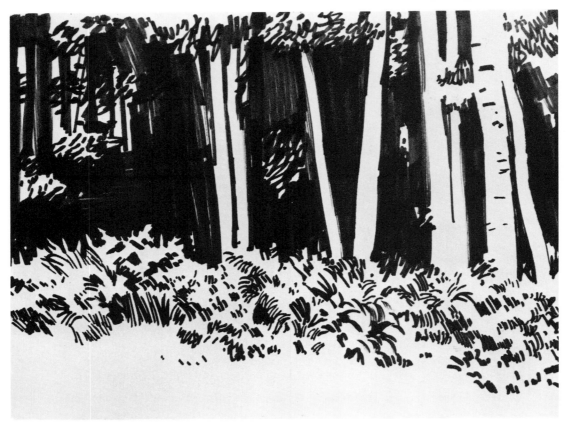

1

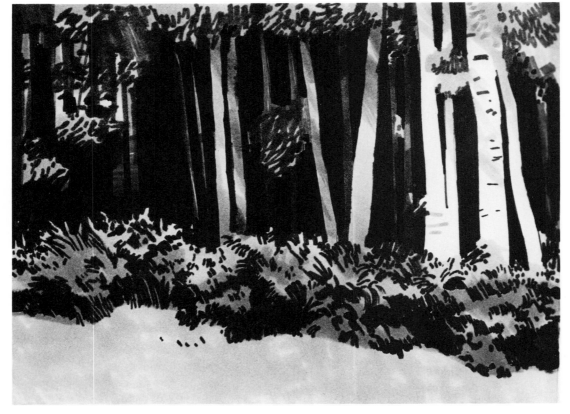

2

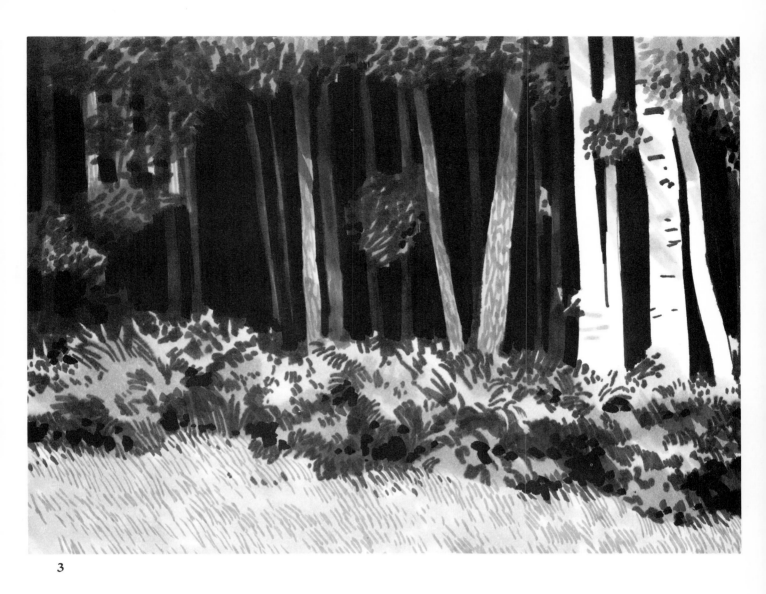

3

Step 1. *Using a No. 7 gray Magic Marker, I block in the darkest background forest area, letting the paper show through where the lighter trees are. In this example, I am departing from my usual procedure of putting in the lighter tones first and then building up the darks. Doing the darks first just turned out to be the easiest way to do this particular picture. After I finish the darks, I put in the shadow areas in the weeds and other foliage in the foreground.*

Step 2. *A light No. 3 gray is added over some of the trees and in the foreground portion. I use a No. 5 gray to put in a few darker tones in the shadows.*

Step 3. *Short marker strokes are put into the foreground to indicate grass. A few more gray tones are added to the foliage, and the shadows are deepened with a No. 9 gray.*

TECHNIQUES

Sunflower: Tone line and tone on synthetic paper.
Nos. 1, 4, 7, and 9 grays were used to paint this sunflower. The basic drawing was done using a Pantone 415F marker. The actual size reproduction at right shows how I cut back into the darker gray tones with the light No. 1 gray, creating an interesting effect.

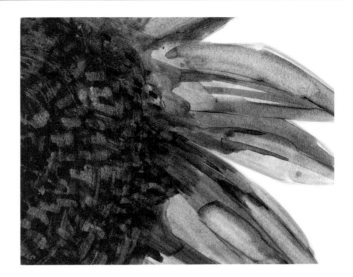

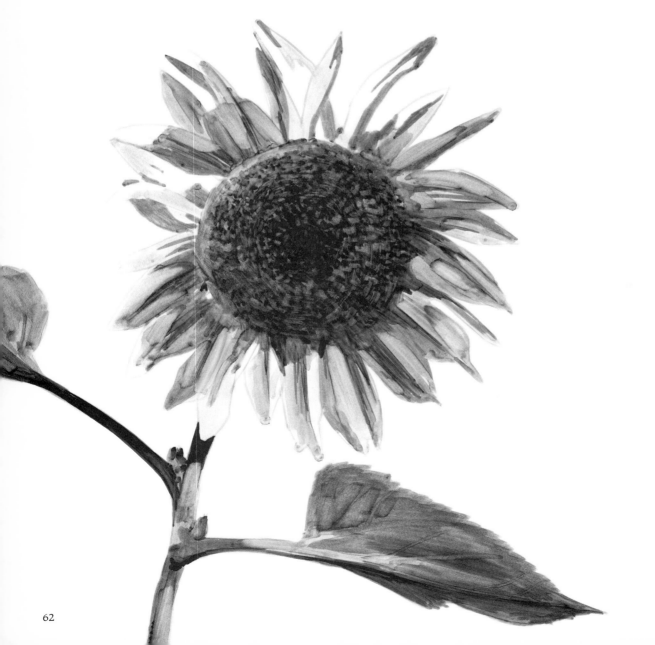

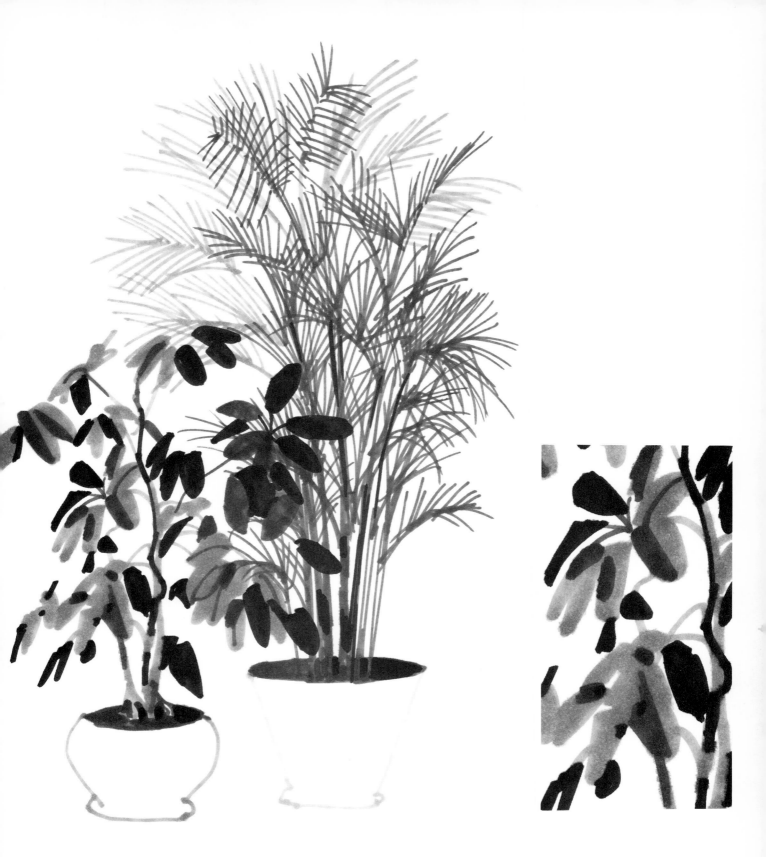

House plants: Bold stroke technique. *These plants were rendered with very fast, bold strokes. The lighter tones were done first, the darks added last. The detail shows how freely the strokes were put down.*

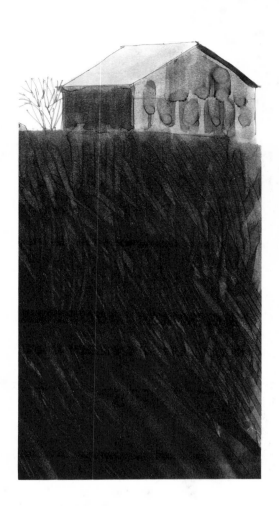

Grasses: Pencil and tone on synthetic paper. *I used 2H pencil to do the basic drawing here and built up the gray tones, from light to dark. The grass texture was put in by using a very light gray marker over the dark background.*

The detail at left shows more clearly how the grass textures were cut back into the darker tone. Notice how—on the barn—the tones dried in a slight blob, creating an interesting effect. When working with markers, don't be afraid of many of the accidental effects and textures that occur. Frequently these accidents add a nice spontaneity to the painting.

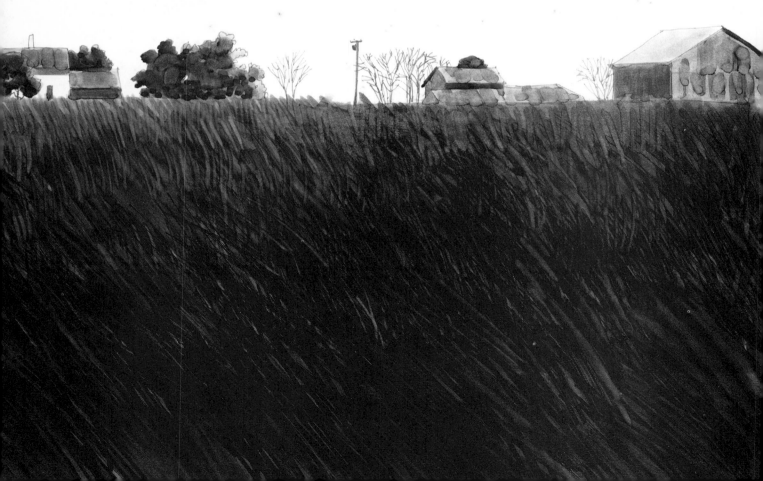

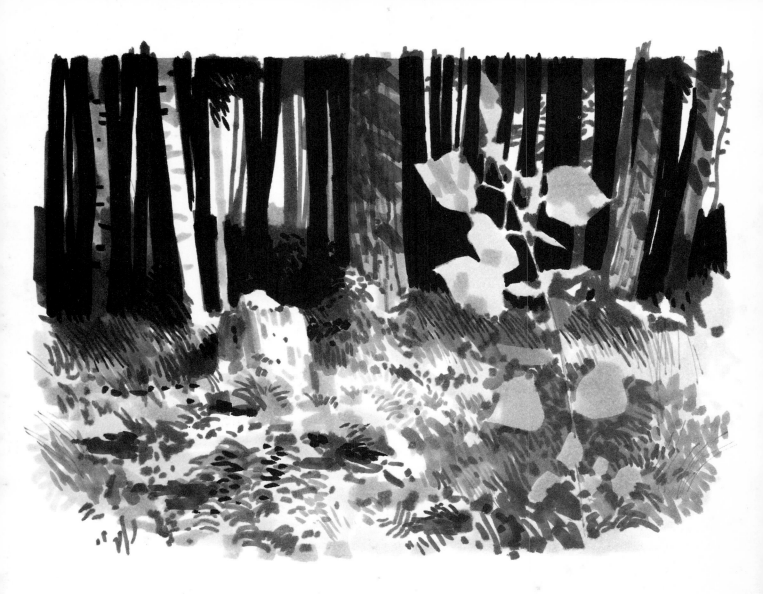

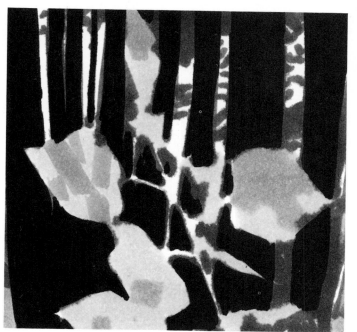

Forest underbrush: Tone on Bristol board.
The lightest tones were put in initially; then the dark tones were added. To achieve the right effect on the foreground plant, I had to render around it. When using markers, you must always carefully plan where the lighter areas will be so you know where to let the paper show through.

On the detail at left, you can see how marker tones soften slightly on Bristol board.

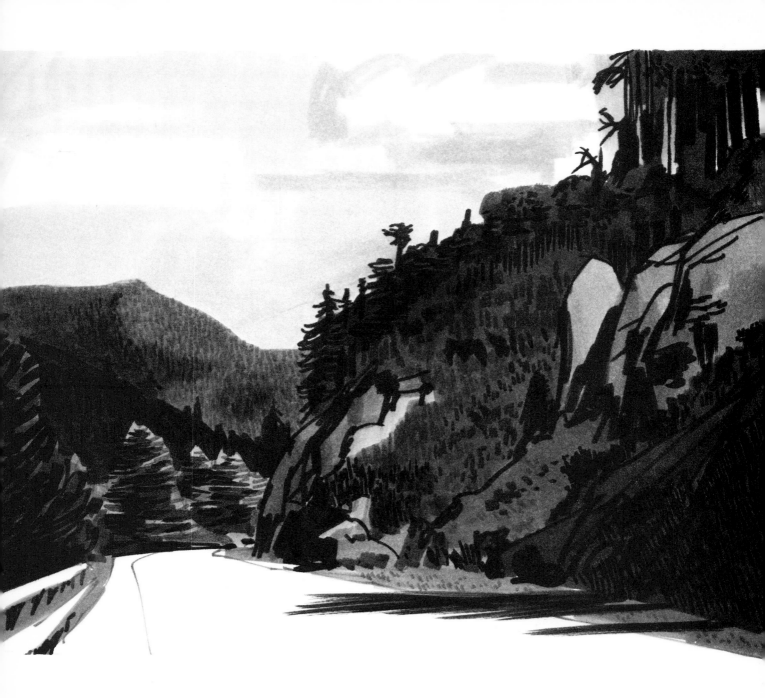

Rocks and hills: Bold stroke technique. *Here I did my basic drawing with a No. 9 gray Magic Marker. The intermediate tones were put in next and the textural detail added over them. The sky was done by opening the marker bottle and drawing directly with the fibrous material that contains the dye.*

CHAPTER FIVE

Rocks and Mountains

ALL LAND FORMS lend themselves well to marker painting techniques. There are many ways to render mountains and rocks—frequently, the best method to begin with is to start by painting in the shadow areas and then building up the intermediate tones. You've got to plan your picture first by drawing small tonal sketches of your subject.

The use of textures and strong shadows is especially important when rendering land forms. Because of this, do your outdoor sketches and paintings either early or late in the day. At this time the sun is lower, casting longer shadows that help emphasize the shapes.

One of the techniques shown in this chapter is an unusual one in which I work with a water-soluble marking pen—then Pentel Sign pen—in combination with a brush and clear water. The Pentel tones dissolve in the water, creating an effect similar to watercolor. Of course, this wash effect can be utilized for many subjects other than land forms.

For painting practice subjects, I suggest—again—that you copy some of my renderings, stroke for stroke. You will see that many of them are really quite simple to do. Remember to try to work in a bold manner, and don't be overly concerned with how the marker goes on the paper surface. It helps to work with fresh, wet markers—save the drier ones for special effects when required.

For finding reference material on mountains, canyons, and all sorts of related subjects, National Geographic and Arizona Highways are very good sources. If you're lucky enough to live in a mountainous region, you have no problem—just go outside and paint.

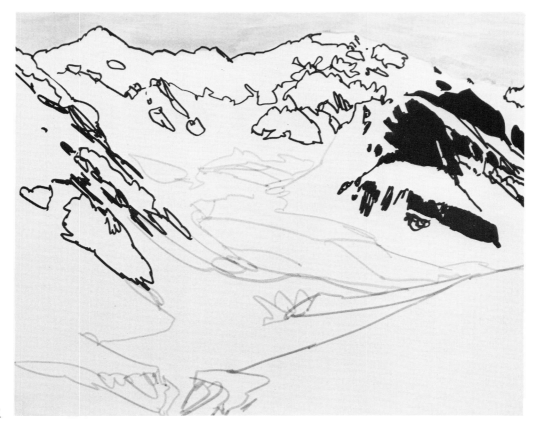

1

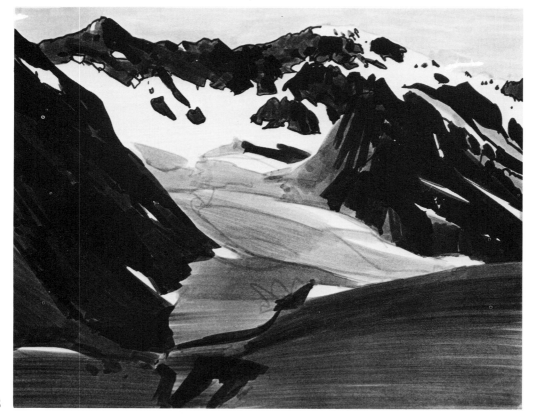

2

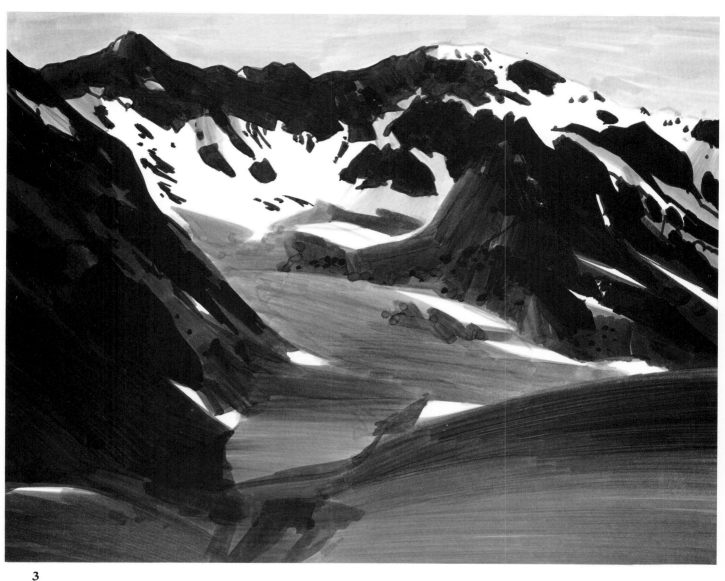

3

Step 1. *I start by carefully drawing in the mountain shapes with a No. 4 gray—the darker lines and tones are added with a No. 9. Then I put a light gray tone into the sky area.*

Step 2. *After I block in the other gray tones using Nos. 5, 7, and 9 grays, I add the darkest black accents.*

Step 3. *The picture is completed by modeling and blending some of the tones in the center of the painting. The initial guidelines I drew were removed by going over the center area with a wet marker. On coated papers, you can usually dissolve unwanted lines in this manner, because the markers don't soak deep into the surface.*

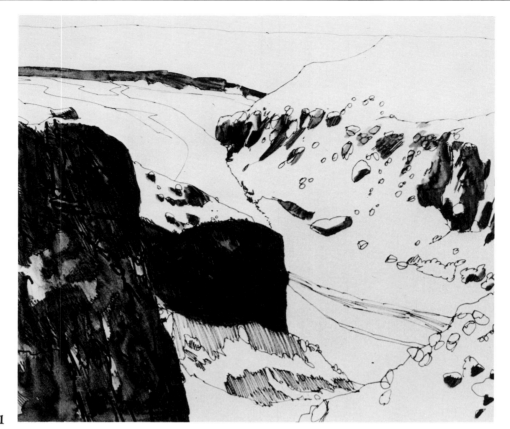

1

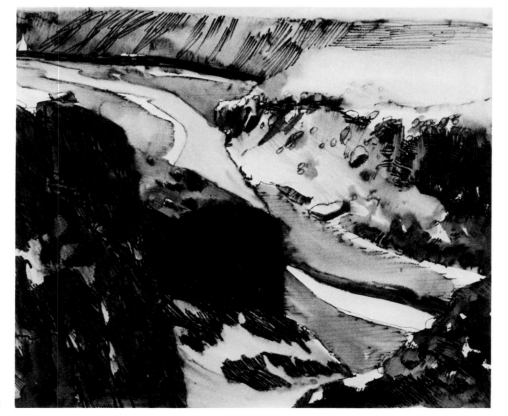

2

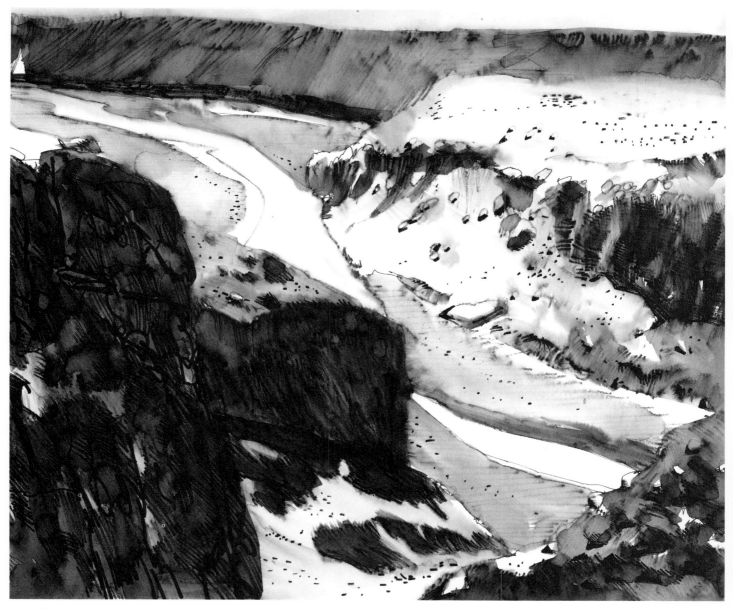

3

Step 1. *In this demonstration, I will show you how to do a painting with a watercolor effect on a sheet of Strathmore regular-surfaced 4-ply board. This is a very good paper surface that I frequently use when doing ink line drawings. First I do a basic drawing with a Pilot Fineliner pen. Then I put in shadow tones with a Pentel Sign pen. I have started to wash clear water over these tones with a large sable brush to dissolve the Pentel, creating a watercolor effect.*

Step 2. *I carefully brush water over most of picture (leaving certain areas white for better contrast), causing the Pentel to dissolve into a very light gray tone. After the washes dry, I add more Pentel lines, darkening some of the tones further. At the top of the picture, at the extreme right middle-ground, and on the foreground cliff, you can see how I continue to shade with the Pentel.*

Step 3. *A few more Pentel tones are added and dissolved with the water. Some of the very dark rock accents were put in with a black Markette pen. This is an excellent technique to use for outdoor sketching, as a minimum of supplies and tools are required—I usually use this method to record scenes when traveling.*

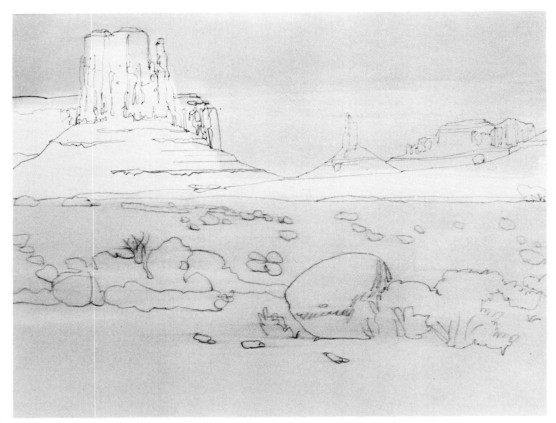

1

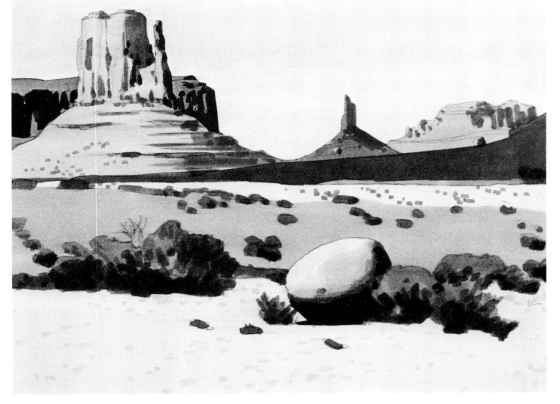

2

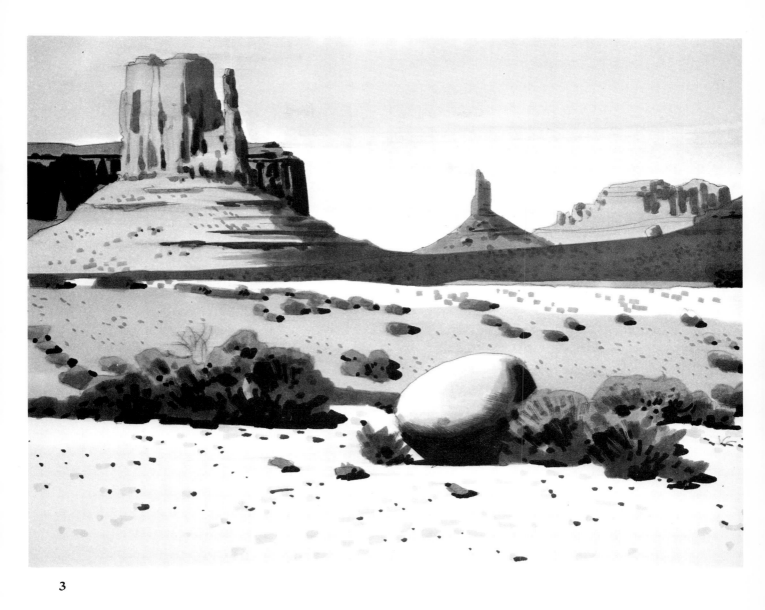

3

Step 1. *I put a No. 2 gray tone over a light pencil drawing. The method I used for painting these rather large gray areas is discussed in detail in Chapter 6. Briefly, I open the Magic Marker bottle, remove the fibrous material, and work directly with it. The fiber can be held with a pair of pliers. It's a sure way to achieve a very smooth tone over a large area.*

Step 2. *I add the other tones carefully, being sure to contrast light and dark tones for an effect of depth. I use Nos. 2, 3, 4, 5, and 9 grays at this point.*

Step 3. *Details, such as the little dots indicating stones and rocks, are put in as well as shadows on the bushes, completing the picture.*

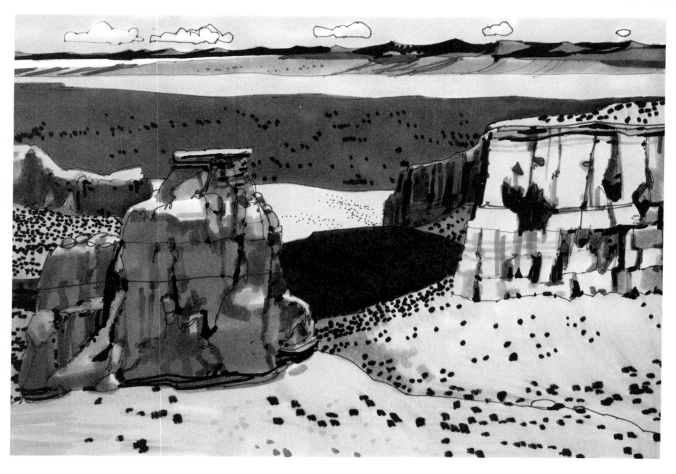

Rock formations: Tone line and tone on Bristol.
The basic drawing was done using a Pantone 417F, after which I added a few light No. 2 gray tones. I built up the picture gradually with darker grays and added the blacks as the finishing touch. The detail at right shows the rather loose, sketchy line I used for my basic drawing.

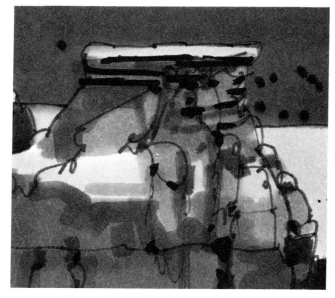

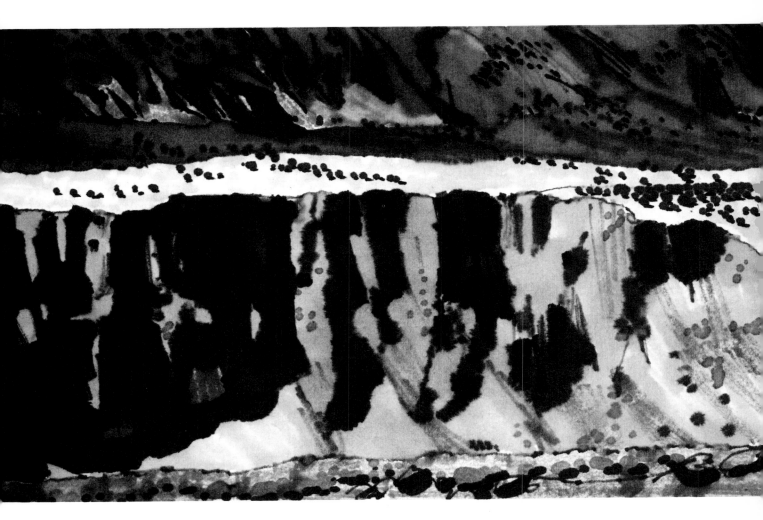

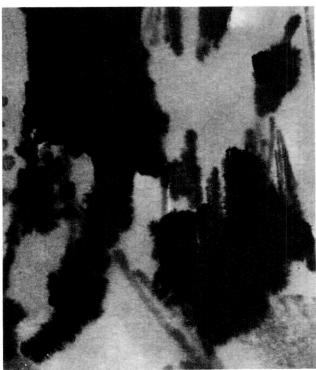

Canyon on rice paper. *Working on a sheet of rice paper, I began this painting by doing a very rough diagram with a Pantone 417F pen. The lightest tones were done first, and then, while the paper was still wet, I added some of the darker values. This caused the tones to blend and spread slightly. Markers used in this manner on rice paper have a distinct watercolor feeling. When you do this, be sure to use a backing sheet, as the markers bleed through the rice paper.*

In the detail at left, you can see more clearly the soft effect created by using the darker markers over the slightly damp surface.

Rock formations on coated paper. *Again, the basic drawing here was done with a Pantone 417F pen. The other areas were built up gradually, and, as in most of the other examples, the darker tones were put in last.*

An actual-size detail showing how the markers go on a coated paper is at right. Note that the tone edges are not as soft as on other surfaces.

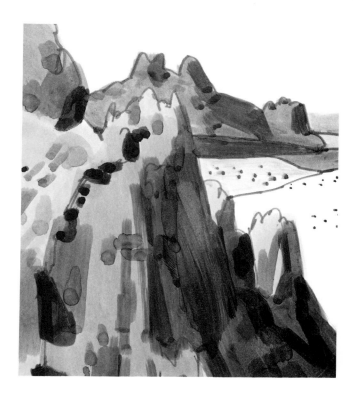

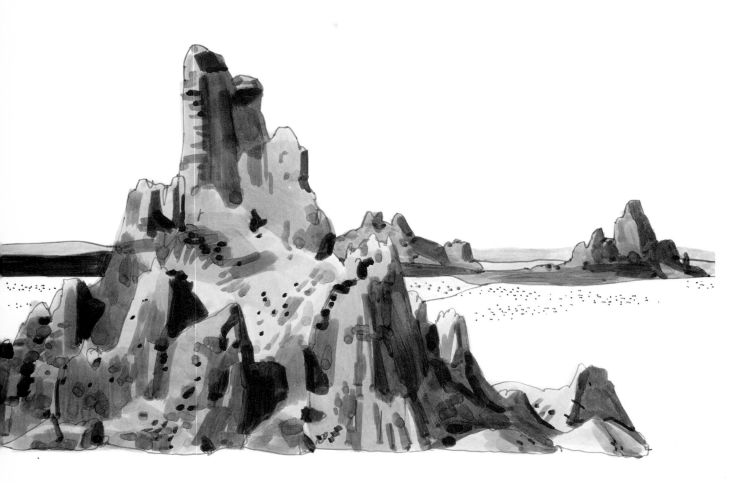

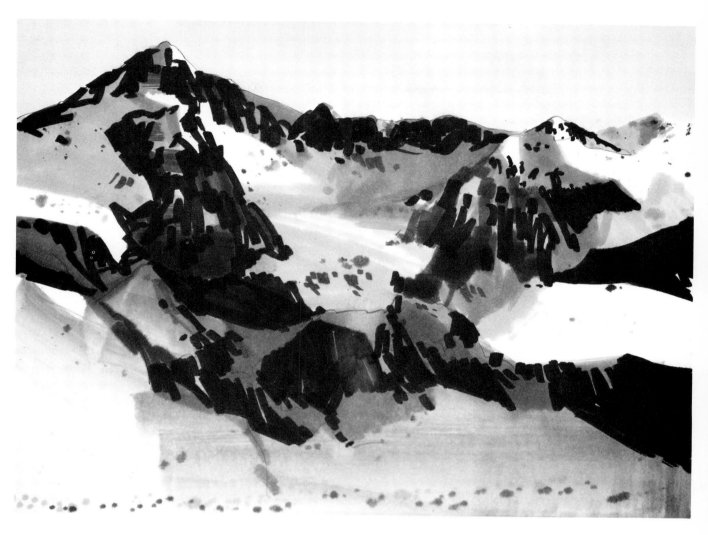

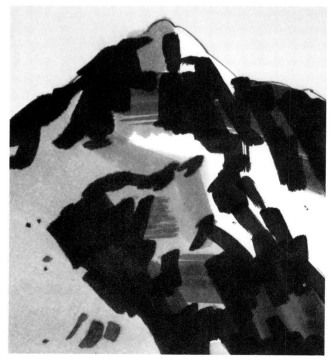

Mountains: Bold stroke technique on Bristol. *I began by drawing a very rough diagram of the scene with a Pantone 417F pen. I added the lighter tones first and then the darker tones, so the effect would be softer through blending. The rendering was finished by adding the Nos. 7 and 9 grays.*

This detail shows the slightly soft effect achieved when working on Bristol. This is a very simple, strong technique. Try not to be timid when using your markers—use bold, direct strokes, as I have done in this example.

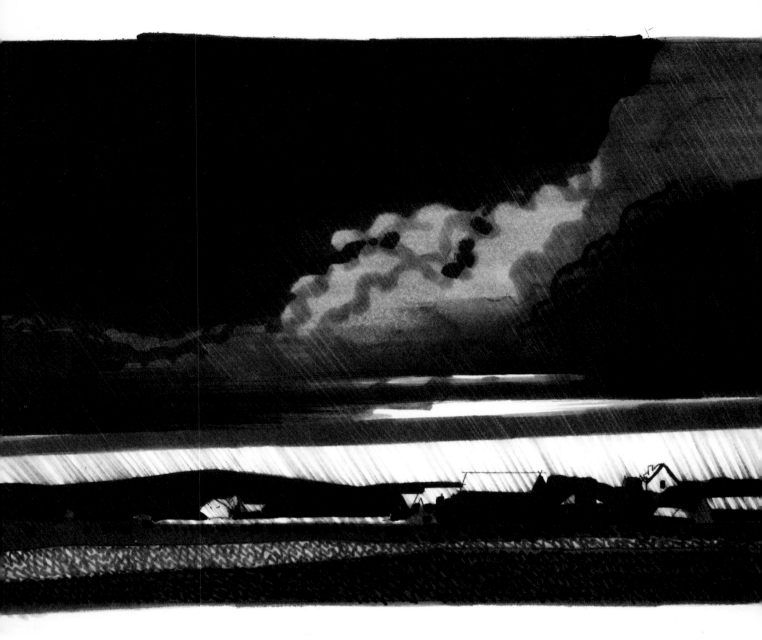

Midwestern rain storm. *This example was first drawn with a pencil on a smooth Bristol board. The tones were added with Nos. 3, 5, 7, and 9 grays and black. The rain effect on the white portion of the sky was achieved by using a fairly dry No. 2 gray marker. Over the dark gray and black areas, I used a Prismacolor white pencil to indicate rain—I kept the pencil point quite sharp so the lines would remain thin throughout. Prismacolor pencils combine very nicely with markers. In Color Demonstration 7, I show how markers and colored pencils can be effectively used together.*

CHAPTER SIX

Skies and Weather

ALL OF THE TECHNIQUES discussed so far are suitable for painting skies and weather conditions. However, one of the most difficult problems encountered when using markers is how to render a perfectly smooth, flat tone. It's very difficult to paint a large, flat sky with markers since the dye dries so quickly. Invariably, the strokes used are quite visible. In one of the demonstrations in this chapter I will show you a perfect method for achieving flat, smooth tones by actually using the inner fibrous core of the Magic Marker to paint with.

Another problem you may encounter is how to paint wispy clouds, which are also quite difficult to render with the normal marker nib. The easiest way to do this is to mix your own colors with Flo-Master inks and brush them on the paper as if you were doing a watercolor. Very soft, blended effects can be accomplished using this method. Rice papers are especially good to use when you paint clouds with regular markers—the markers tend to blend on rice paper, resulting in watercolor effects.

Many times when a certain effect is impossible with markers, Prismacolor or similar pencils can be used over them. You can even use white paint, but keep it to a minimum so the painting does not look overworked.

DEMONSTRATION 11. PAINTING A FLAT SKY

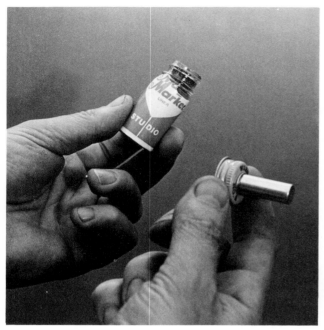

Step 1. *When a large, flat, smooth tone is desired, it is most easily accomplished by using this method with Magic Marker Studio markers. You can uncap the container, remove the inner fibrous core that contains the color, and use it for painting.*

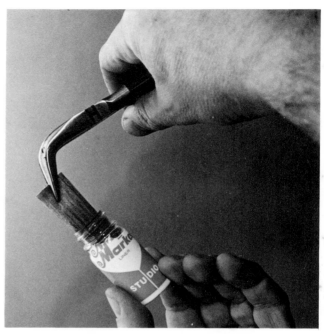

Step 2. *Using a needle-nosed plier, I remove the inner core. (Please note that you can wear gloves if you like although I don't.) It's best to remove it this way so your fingers do not become stained by the dye.*

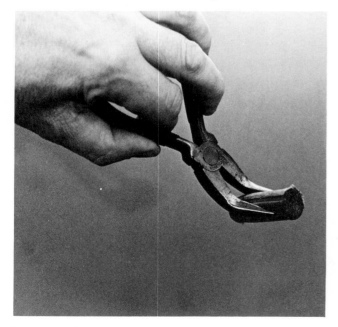

Step 3. *I hold the core as shown, keeping a firm grip on the pliers.*

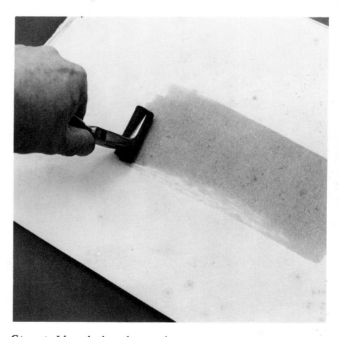

Step 4. *I brush the color on the paper surface using quick, bold strokes. When the color dries, I have a perfectly smooth tone that could not be achieved with the normal marker nib.*

DEMONSTRATION 12. PAINTING CLOUDS WITH A BRUSH AND DYES

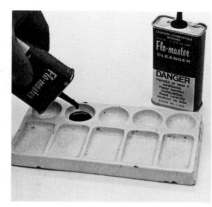

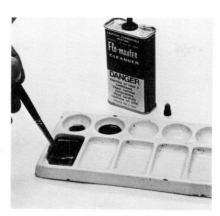

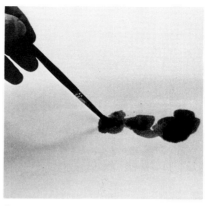

Step 1. *I put a few drops of the Flo-master black transparent ink in a ceramic tray.*

Step 2. *In another well, I pour some Flo-master cleanser (solvent). Using a brush, I dilute a little of the black to get a gray tone.*

Step 3. *I dampen a piece of Aquabee plate-finish Bristol using the solvent and a paper towel. When the paper surface is quite wet, I start to brush on some of the diluted ink.*

Step 4. *(Top) I add some lighter gray tones by further diluting the black ink. Note that I make no attempt to actually blend the tones. The blending and softness occur because the paper is still damp from the solvent. A nice, soft cloud effect can be easily achieved using this method. Be very careful not to overwork your subject when using this technique.*

(Above) A very odd but interesting cloud effect happened on the other side of the paper because of bleed-through. Often you can utilize such an effect and incorporate it in a painting. Occasionally, what happens on the other side of the paper proves to be more interesting than what you were trying to do. (Because of this tendency for the dyes to bleed through, always use a backing sheet.)

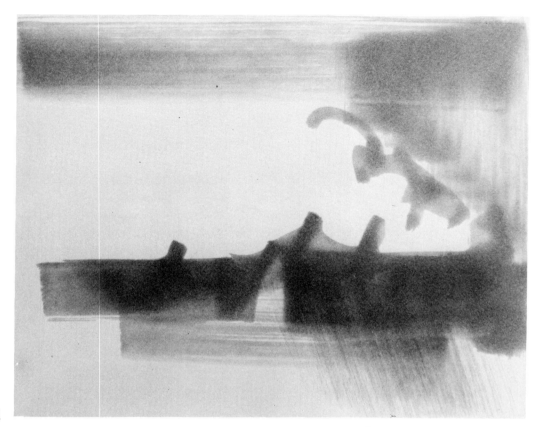

1

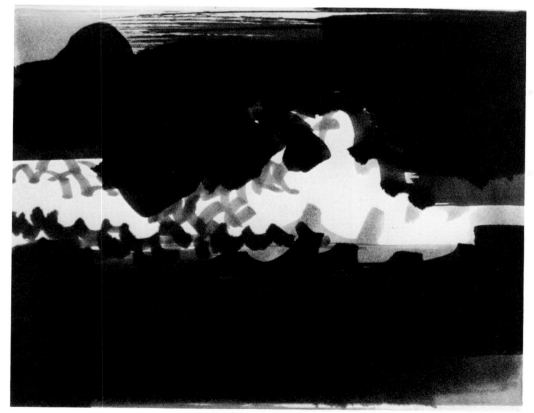

2

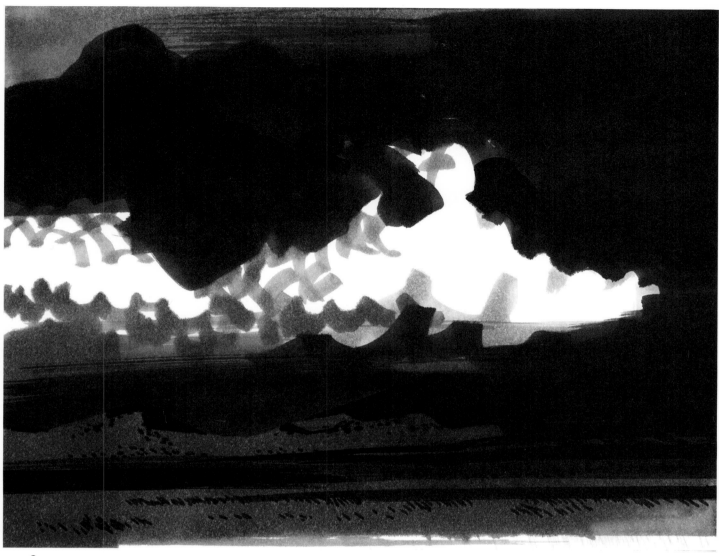

3

Step 1. *After removing the inner core of the Magic Marker No. 4 gray, I start painting in the tones on the Aquabee plate-finish Bristol board with very bold strokes, holding the core firmly with needle-nosed pliers.*

Step 2. *While the paper is still a little damp from the first tone, I work over the picture with a No. 5 gray. Then, removing the core from a No. 7 gray, I add more darks to the scene.*

Step 3. *Cloud details are added with a No. 7 and a black Magic Marker with the normal marker nib. I add shadows to form the hills and mountains with the black marker and a few textures and foreground tones with a No. 7 gray.*

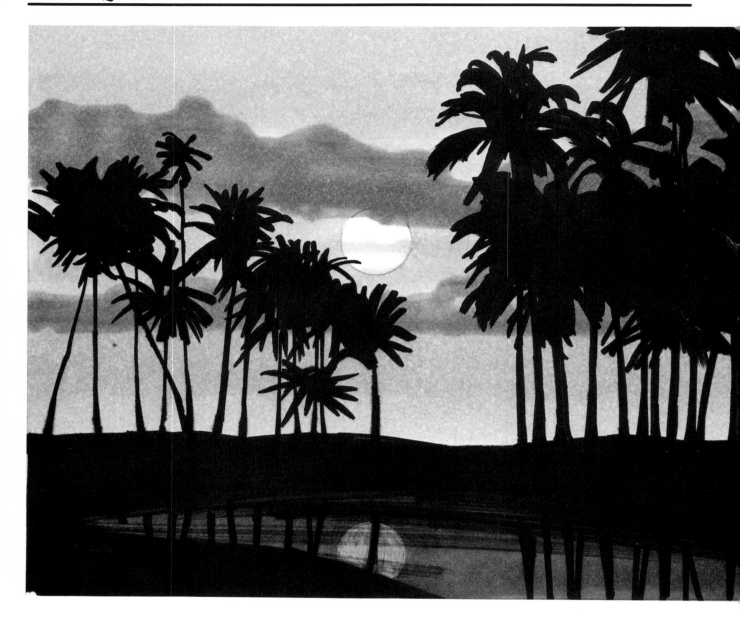

Dusk. *(Above) Frequently at the end of the day when the sun is low, everything is reduced to a flat tone or silhouette without much form. This dusk scene was done using only Nos. 2 and 5 gray with black for the trees. When you do sketches and paintings like this, try to think in simple terms like I did here. Note that the reflection of the sun in the pool was done with a white Prismacolor pencil.*

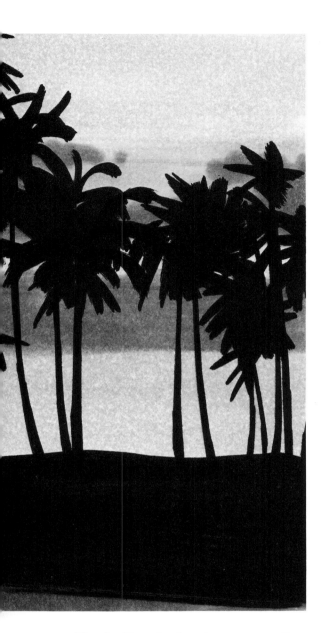

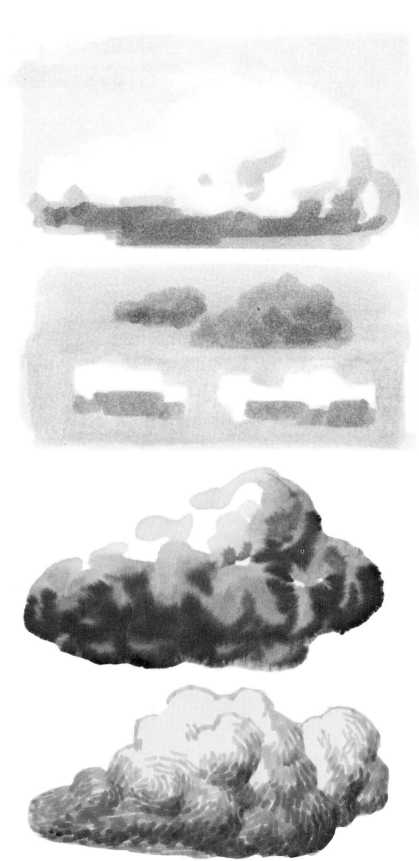

Clouds. *Top, clouds on layout paper. Center, cloud done by using bold marker strokes to achieve a better illusion of form. When doing objects in this style, you should make the strokes follow the shape to help mold the form. Three grays were used here on a smooth Bristol board. Bottom, cloud on rice paper. When working over previously done tones, you get a blended effect.*

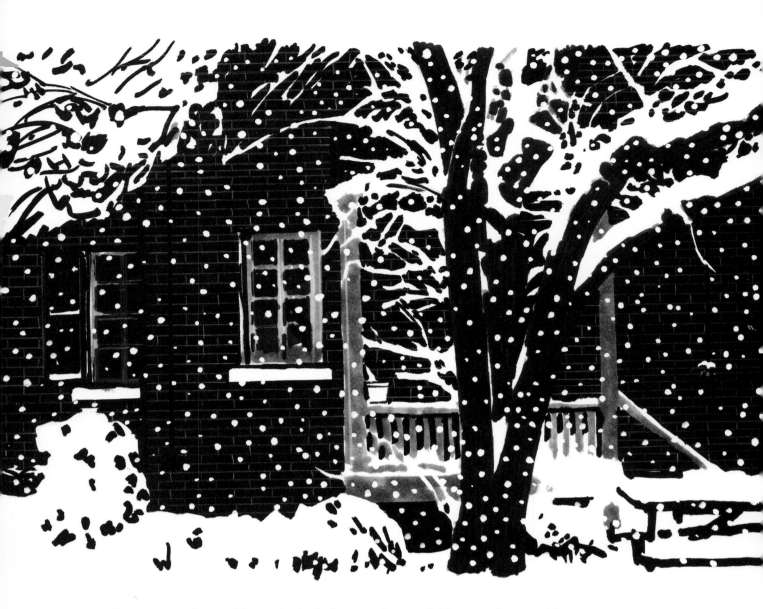

Snow scene. *I started by putting in the house and tree with Nos. 7 and 9 grays. Nos. 3 and 4 grays were used on the porch and windows. I carefully let the white paper show through in the right areas to indicate the snow and drew in the bricks with a white Prismacolor pencil. I added the snowflakes last with white paint and a brush.*

CHAPTER SEVEN

Water, Snow, and Ice

MOST PAPERS and techniques work well for these subjects, although you may encounter some problems because of insufficient planning. White areas—such as snow, whitecaps, and reflections—must be carefully planned through sketches. When working in paint, you can simply paint white areas back in; but when working with markers, you can't do this. You must utilize the white paper.

Study the examples in this chapter carefully—many have been broken down into two or three simple tone values. Always try to keep your work simple, especially when doing fast sketches. Markers can be overworked, and, when this happens, you have lost your painting and must start over. If you start to overwork a painting, most probably you have not planned it properly. But if you try to solve as many problems as possible in the preliminary sketch stage, you will save yourself a lot of grief and paper.

Start to collect a picture file of water, rivers, ocean waves, and snow scenes—this reference material can prove invaluable when you are confronted with a difficult rendering problem.

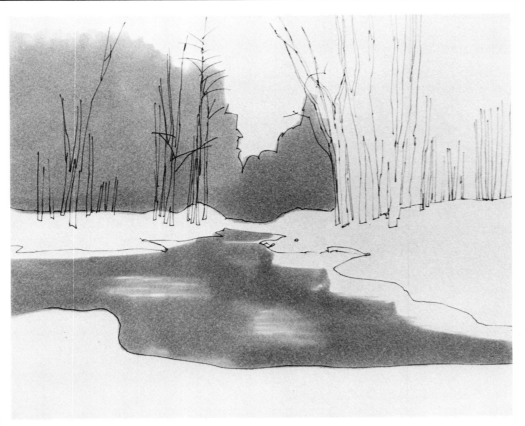

1

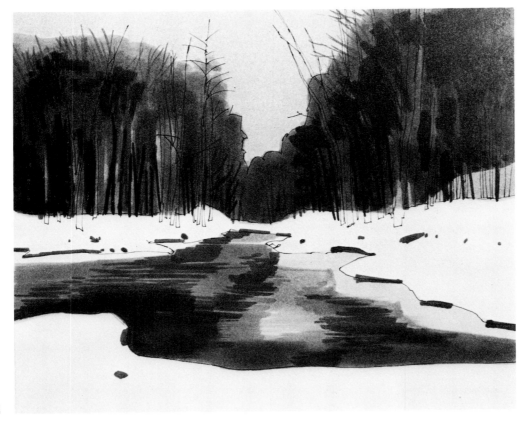

2

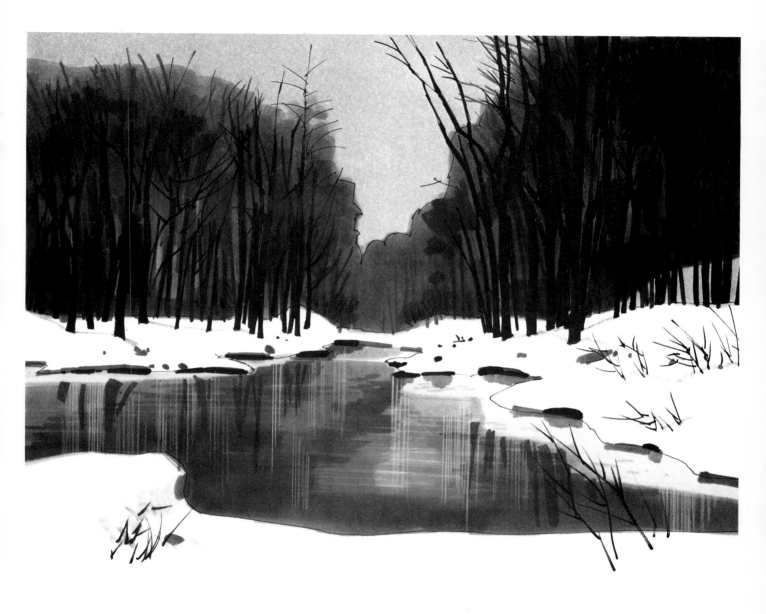

3

Step 1. *I start by doing a diagramatic drawing on smooth Bristol with a Niji Stylist pen, establishing the first tones with a No. 4 gray marker.*

Step 2. *With a No. 2 gray marker, I put in the sky, going over the area a few times to even out the tone. When working on a plate-finish Bristol, tones can be easily smoothed out in this manner, although the gray value will be somewhat darker if you add a gray tone over the same gray. Next, I start to add the dark tones to the trees and darken some of the ice with a No. 7 gray. I go over the whole background with a No. 5 gray, and add a few darker tones with the No. 7. The tree trunks are darkened with a No. 9 gray.*

Step 3. *More trees are added to the background with a black Markette Thinrite pen. Then the brushes and twigs in the foreground are added with the same pen. Reflections on the ice made with a white Eagle Prismacolor pencil plus a few tree reflections complete the picture.*

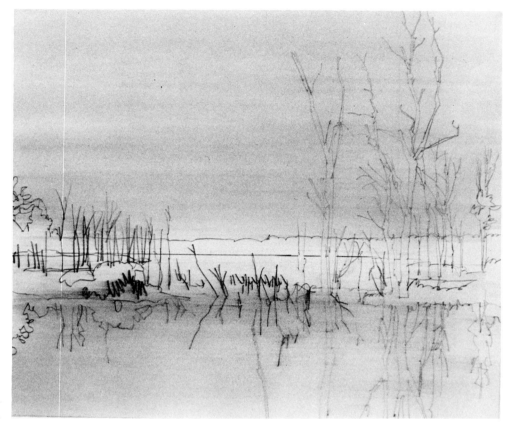

1

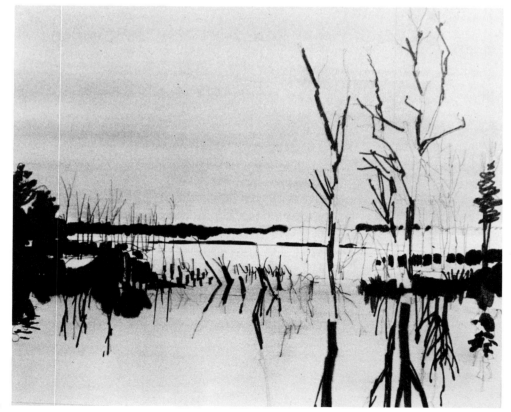

2

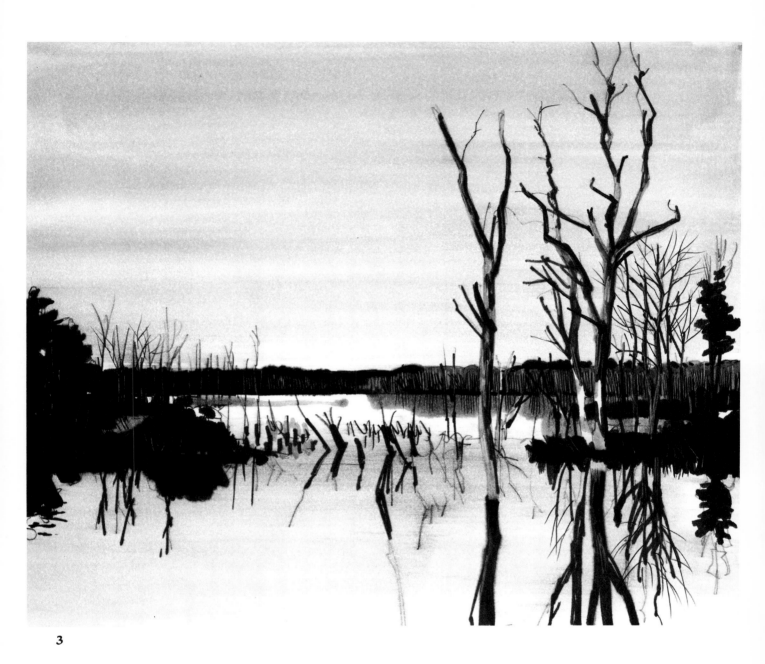

3

Step 1. *I start by doing a rough—but accurate—pencil drawing with an HB grade pencil on smooth Bristol board. The sky tone is done with a No. 2 gray, using the inner core of the Magic Marker as shown in Demonstration 11. I go over the water area with the No. 2 gray also. Note that the marker slightly smears the pencil drawing, creating an interesting effect.*

Step 2. *With a No. 7 gray, I start to add darker foreground areas and tones on the trees. The reflections in the water are done using the same gray.*

Step 3. *I add a No. 3 gray to the background and to the tree trunks in the foreground. Then I continue to work on the trees with a No. 5 gray. A black marker is used for accents throughout the picture, and a white Prismacolor pencil to bring out the twigs and background trees. This painting consists of only four tones, Nos. 3, 5, and 7 grays and black.*

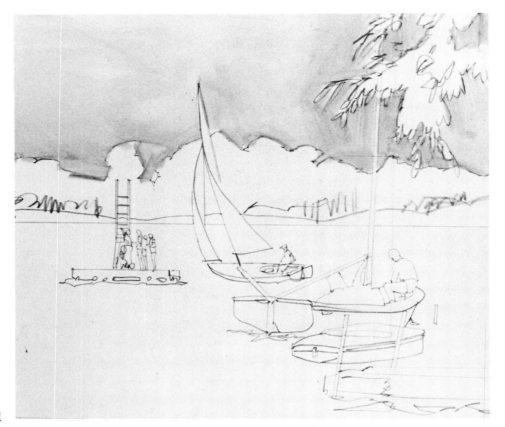

1

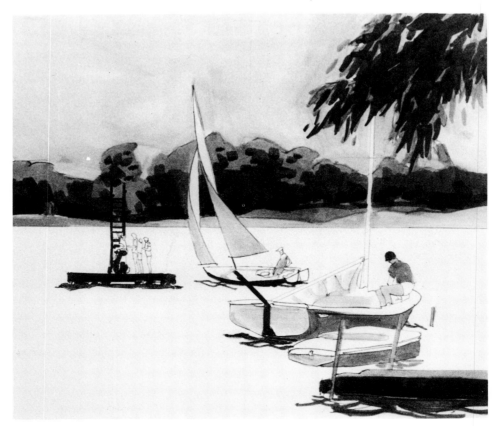

2

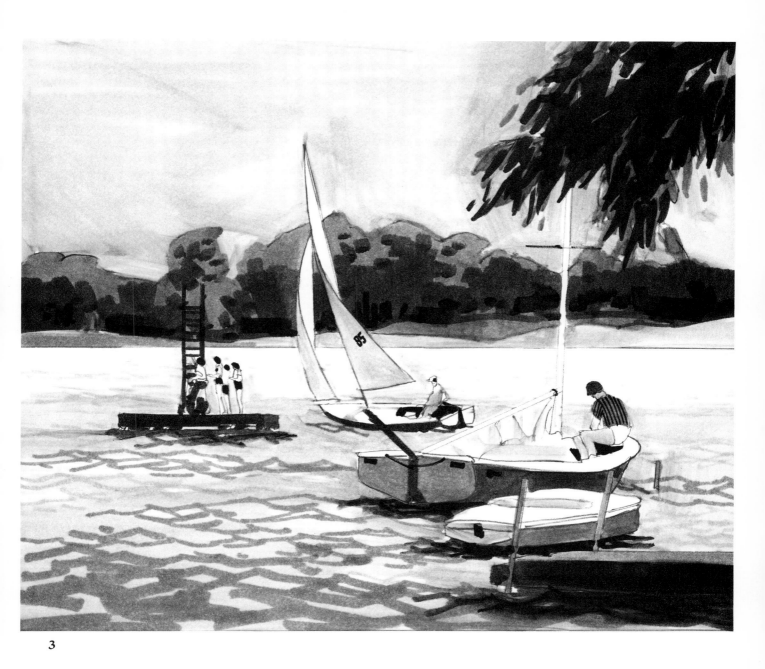

3

Step 1. *I first do a pencil drawing on layout paper and add a sky tone with a No. 2 gray marker.*

Step 2. *I put shadow tones in the background trees with a No. 7 gray. The shadows of the boats are also done with that gray. Next, the waves and the leaves are indicated with a No. 2 gray, the very dark tones being put in with a No. 9. A No. 7 intermediate tone is added to the background trees.*

Step 3. *I put a No. 2 gray on the foreground water area and draw a No. 4 gray wave texture over this. Using a No. 1 gray, I do the background water area. Finally, I darken the shadows and add black accents.*

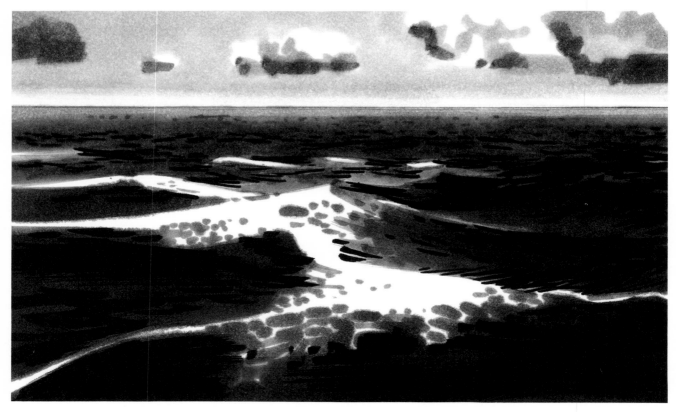

Ocean waves. *This is a fairly simple rendering of a complex subject. The sky is done with Nos. 2 and 3 grays, the clouds with Nos. 3, 4, and 5 grays. The water consists of Nos. 3, 4, 5, and 7 grays with a No. 9 gray for the darkest accents. I carefully let enough white paper show through in the proper places to achieve the whitecap effect.*

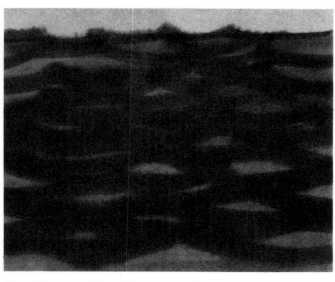

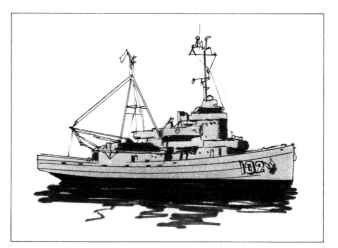

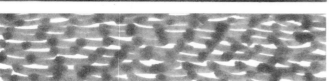

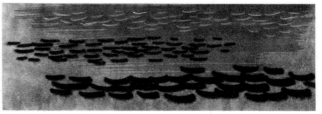

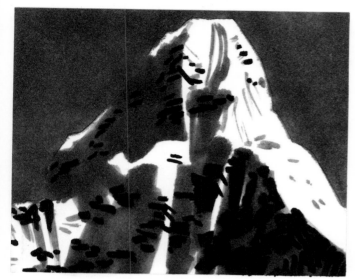

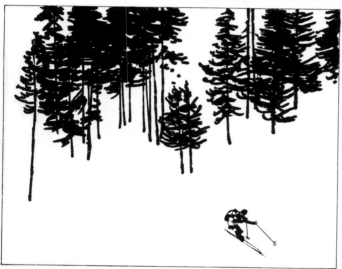

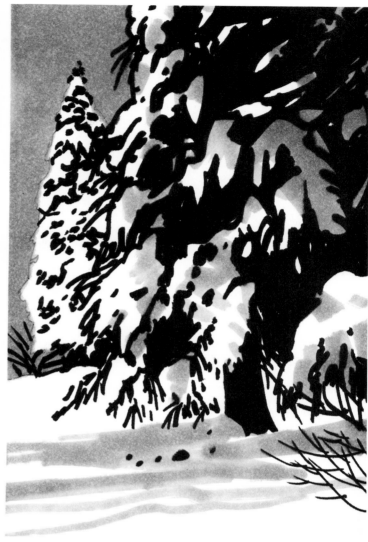

Water. *(Left) Here are a few ways to indicate water: top left, placing one tone over another using curved wavelike strokes—the darker tone is softened because of the slight blending that occurs when using markers on Bristol; bottom left, covering an area with textured strokes, letting a little white show through; top right, putting in only the reflection of the ship—the irregularity of the reflection helps give the impression of water; bottom right, stroking black or dark gray (or even white Prismacolor pencil) over a tone.*

Mountains, trees, and snow. *(Above) Upper left, mountain done using only a No. 5 gray and black. Keep thinking in simple terms like this when rendering objects. Bottom left, snow scene done using only black. Right, scene done with two gray tones, Nos. 3 and 9. It's good to think in very graphic terms when doing sketches—try to think of your scene as a "drop-out" photograph, where the emphasis is on the important shapes and shadows and the rest drops out in white.*

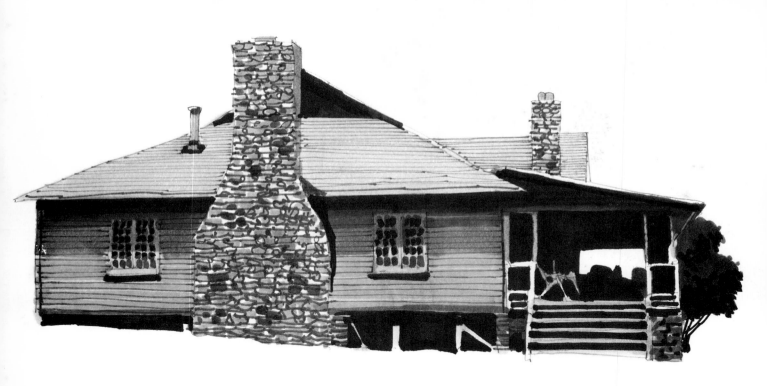

Cabin: Tone on Bristol board. *The flat tones in this example were put over a light pencil drawing. The textures, wood siding, and fireplace (see detail) were accented with a Pantone 417 F fine-line marker.*

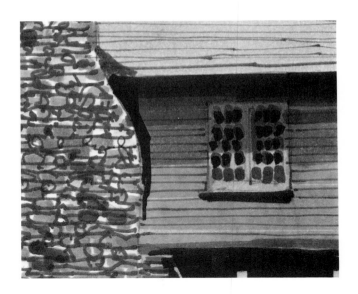

CHAPTER EIGHT

Architectural Subjects

MARKER PAINTINGS of architectural subjects are generally more successful when tone is used in conjunction with line. Because of the nature of the felt nib, it can be difficult to paint very fine details, but it isn't as hard to use line. On involved subjects, such as ornate churches, the use of line to bring out detail is especially helpful.

When first attempting architecture subjects you should work from photographs. You can take your own photos or find good subject matter in magazines. Carefully study the photographs and look at the different kinds of textures that the various building materials have. Wood, brick, and other building material textures are a very important aspect when rendering most architectural subjects. Certain strokes and marks can be produced with the markers that will simulate these materials. Study the examples both in this chapter and in other photos and practice duplicating the textures.

For your basic drawing, you may want to use a ruler or triangle for straight lines. You can sketch very light lines with a pencil, and then use a ruler or triangle to draw the final straight lines. However, buildings need not be done mechanically, as shown in *City* on page 107. As you develop, try working freehand.

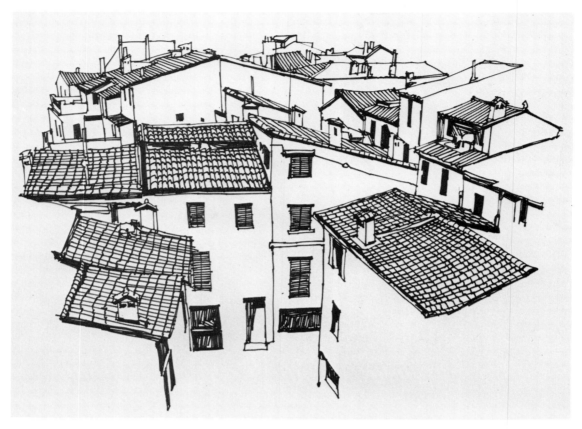

1

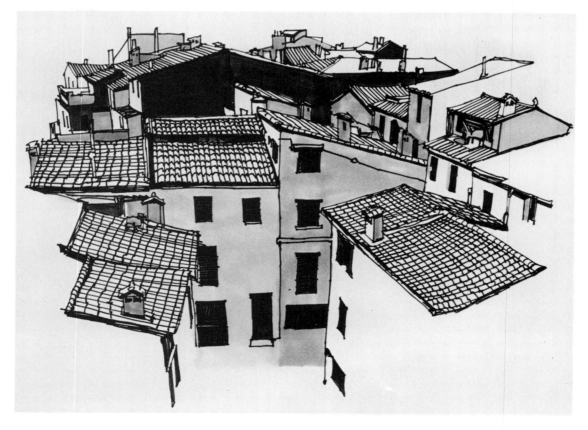

2

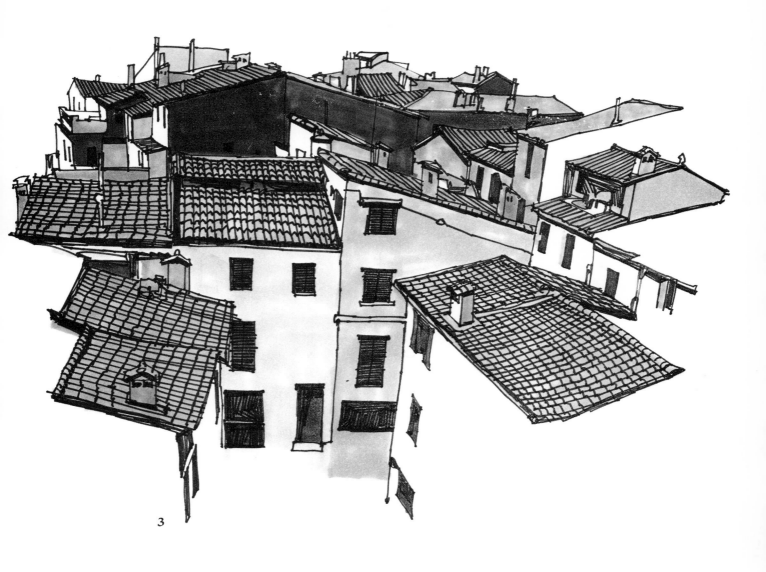

3

Step 1. *The basic drawing is done with a Pantone black fine-line marker. Then I add a few grays to the roof tiles.*

Step 2. *I continue to fill in areas with the Magic Marker grays, keeping aware of the source of light so the shadows are in the correct places.*

Step 3. *The final gray tones are put on the roofs and the rendering is complete. This is a simple, fast technique that can be used for many architectural subjects. You can use markers, pens, or pencils for your basic line drawing; then, as I have done here, simply fill in the gray or color tones to complete the painting. Practice your first architectural painting using this method, as it's one of the easiest.*

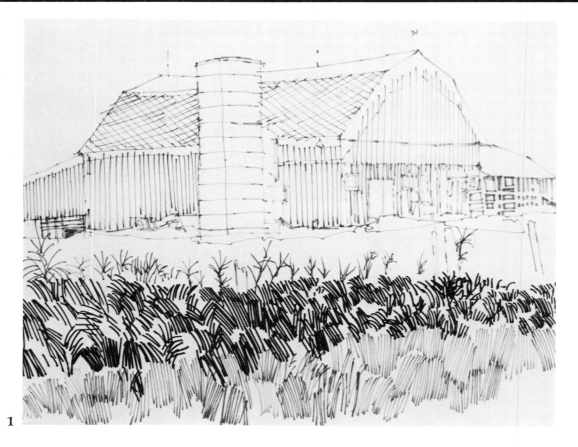

1

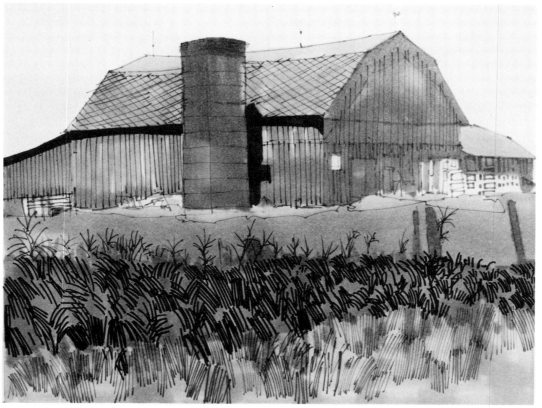

2

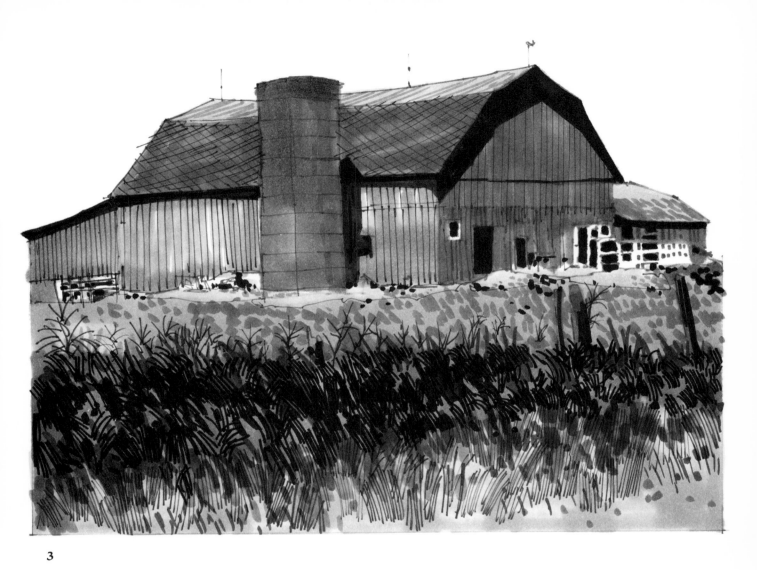

3

Step 1. *First I do a drawing of the barn with a Pantone 415F pen and then I draw some of the foreground foliage with a Pantone 417F. Next a Pantone black fine-line marker is used to put in the darker grass texture.*

Step 2. *The tones are put in with Nos. 2, 3, 5 and 7 grays. On the side of the barn, I use bold downward strokes, leaving a few white streaks showing through to add to the feeling of wood.*

Step 3. *The shadows on the barn are put in with Nos. 7 and 9 grays, and these same tones are added to the foreground grass area. The detail shows the wood effect on the side of the barn.*

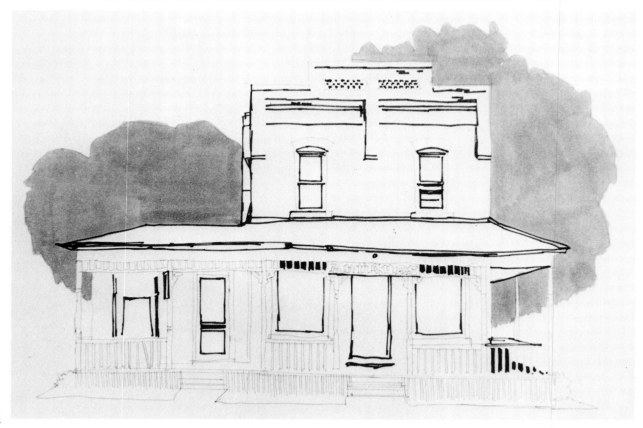

1

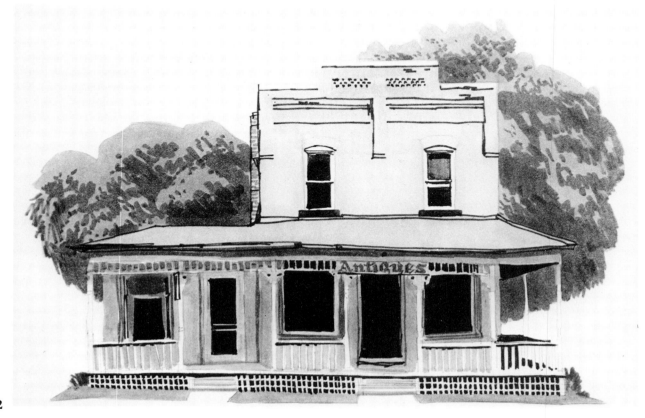

2

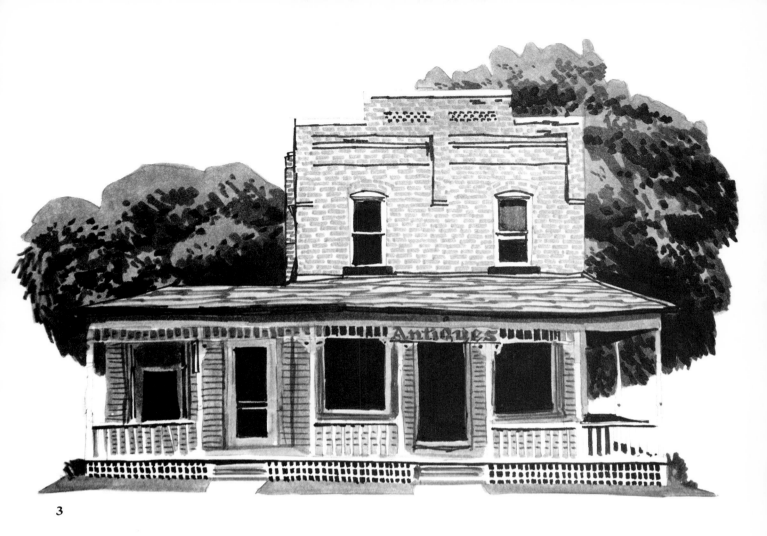

3

Step 1. *To do the drawings of the antique shop, I use an HB grade pencil. After I put in some of the heavier shadow accent lines with a Pantone black fine-line marker, I begin adding gray tones in the background trees.*

Step 2. *The intermediate gray areas are filled in carefully, and some of the shadow tones are put on the trees.*

Step 3. *The building is finished by adding a brick texture carefully with the edge of the marker nib. The lines on the roof, indicating shingles, are done last.*

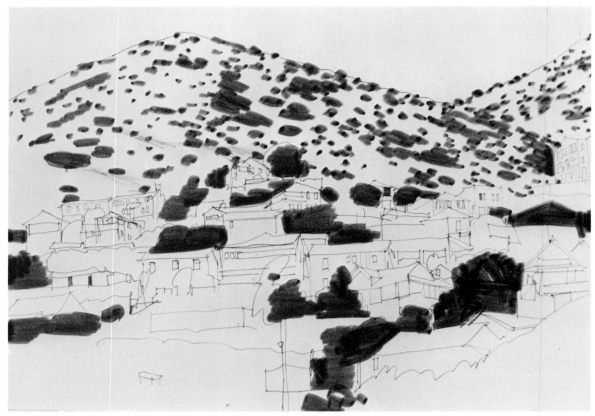

1

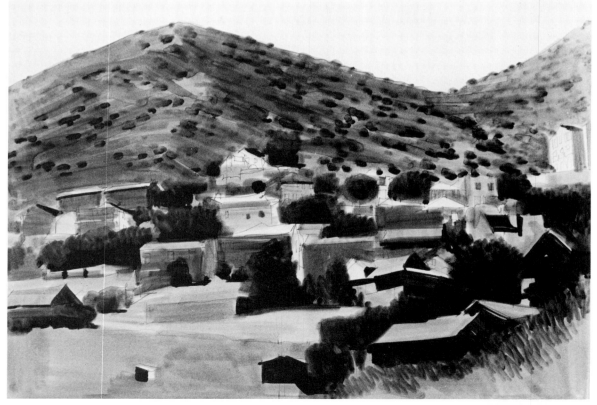

2

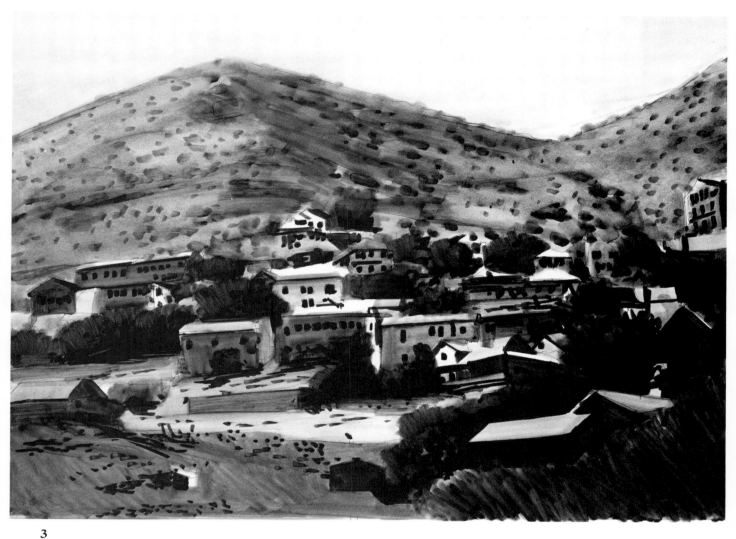

3

Step 1. *I start this painting by first doing a fast dia-gramatic sketch of the buildings and hills with an HB grade pencil. Next I put a medium gray tone on the foliage on the hills and in the foreground.*

Step 2. *I gradually build up the intermediate and darker tones, being careful to leave some white paper showing through where I want highlighted accents.*

Step 3. *The background hill is reworked a little by cutting into the dark tones with a No. 1 gray. Because the markers don't soak in very much on this synthetic paper, Kimdura, it's possible to rework portions of the painting.*

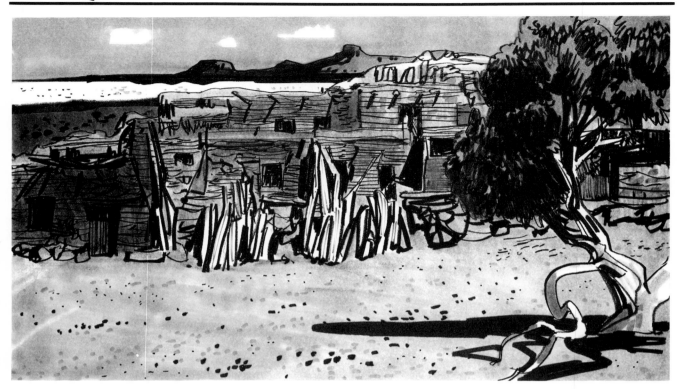

Hopi Indian village: Underdrawing technique.
Charcoal pencil used as a underdrawing is an effective technique for many architectural subjects. I drew this one on a plate-finish Bristol, which takes charcoal very nicely. I sprayed my finished drawing with a little fixative to minimize smudging and then added the gray tones, leaving a few whites to give the scene a little sparkle. The dark shadows and a few tone textures were put in the building last. Some dots and strokes were added to the ground area to suggest shadows of stones and rocks. This is a fast, strong-looking style, but remember that the underdrawing must be very accurate for the method to work successfully. The detail at right shows how few grays were used in this picture.

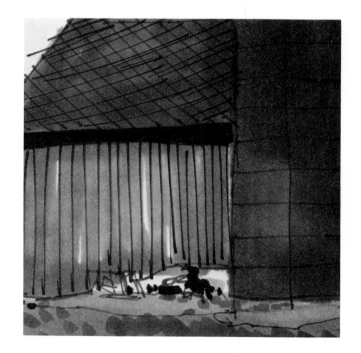

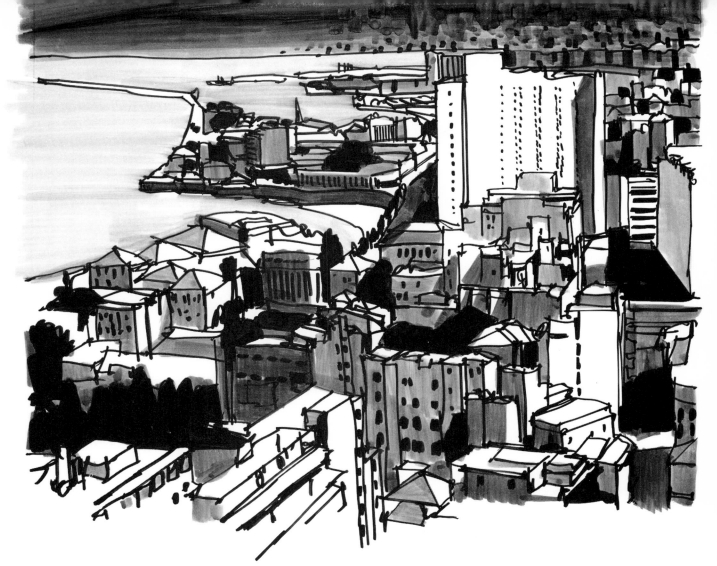

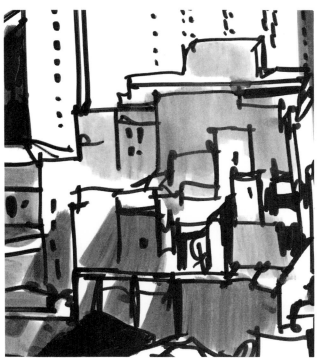

City: Marker line and tone on coated paper. *Buildings and other similar subjects can be handled in a very loose, free style. For this technique to work well, your drawing must be basically correct and the looseness must be the same, generally, over the whole picture.*

Here I first did a very quick, but accurate, drawing of the city using a Markette pen. Then I added the shadows in the proper spots as well as the intermediate grays to help separate the buildings. The distant buildings are put in last. You will learn a great deal if you do many practice studies and sketches using this technique. The coated paper is quite slick, enabling you to work very fast. Working this way can help you to think fast and to learn to see the important parts of a scene quickly.

You can see how loosely the lines were actually drawn from the detail at left.

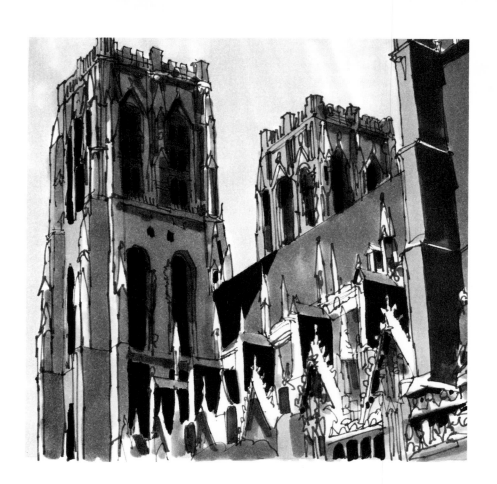

Architectural details. *These two examples clearly demonstrate the importance of line when doing architectural studies with markers. It's almost impossible to put in fine, crisp details, and line can help a great deal. Notice how much more detailed and accurate the top sketch looks.*

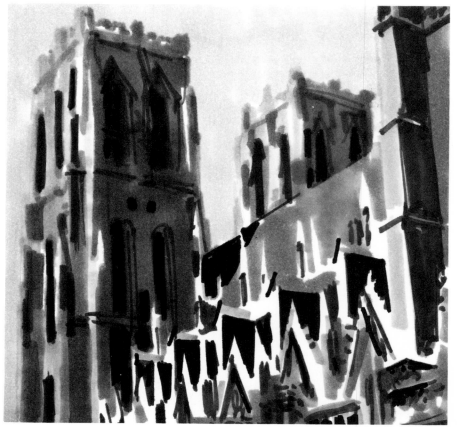

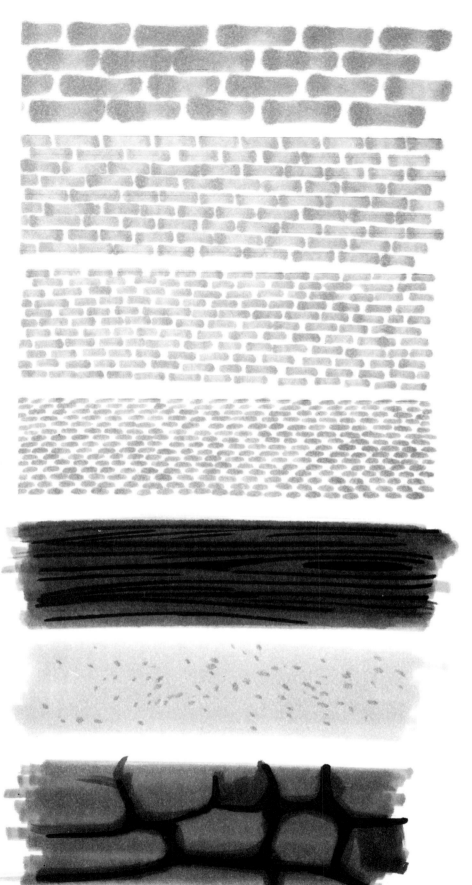

Architectural textures done with a Magic Marker nib. *From top to bottom, four brick sizes were all done using the standard Magic Marker nib, showing how well this versatile nib is designed; a rough wood texture; a fairly smooth cement surface; and large rocks.*

CHAPTER NINE

Demonstrations in Color

THE COLOR DEMONSTRATIONS I have chosen for this chapter incorporate various techniques as well as diverse subject matter. The paintings are shown at various stages of completion to demonstrate clearly how they were done. Study each step and the finished paintings carefully, and try to duplicate them yourself to help you understand them better. You will see how simple some of them are. You don't have to use the same type of paper, but do follow the sequence of steps. Then try some of your own scenes from scratch, using photographs as reference. As you become more familiar with this medium, move on to doing sketches and paintings directly from nature.

In these demonstrations, you will notice that I always build up my dark tones very slowly in order to not overwork areas and get the values too deep. Also, my preliminary planning and basic drawing is always worked out very thoroughly before I start to work in color. I always research my subject matter completely and try to solve most of the problems by doing preliminary sketches.

USING COLOR

With so many marker colors available, the choice of a basic palette can be very confusing. Setting up a color palette with markers is quite different from the palette you would use for watercolor or other paints. You cannot dilute the standard marker colors—as you can regular paints—with water or white paint. This means that you must have a greater number of lighter colors in your basic palette—you can always darken these lighter colors by using grays or other colors over them.

I generally use warm and cool reds, blues, and greens in my palette. For instance, vermilion is a hot red, while crimson is a cooler red. Pale olive is a good warm green, and blue-green is cool. Certain darker colors, such as teal blue, mariner blue, olive, and leather, can be very useful. Be sure to include a pale blue as well as a few other lighter colors that would be impossible to mix.

COLOR PALETTES

My basic color palette is shown in the top row of the chart on the following page. There are 18 colors, 5 grays, and black. With these 18 basic colors, you can mix many other ones by using the colors over one another. The middle row shows some of the color possibilities when these basic colors are mixed. The bottom row shows some of the colors created by mixing grays with the basic colors in the top row.

My marker color palette is not one that I planned—it just developed by itself. I always seem to be running out of the same colors, and these obviously are the ones I use the most. After analyzing several of my paintings and sketches that were done over a long span of time, I realized that there are certain colors I usually work with. My palette is composed of about 24 colors, including gray and black. With these colors I am able to render just about any subject. With 24 colors and grays, you have quite an extensive palette—and these colors can be mixed, creating even more colors. Combining the colors and the grays extends the range even further. The color chart on page 113 shows the great variety of colors possible using this basic palette.

The top row on the chart shows the basic colors and grays I generally use. The center row of colors is produced by mixing together two of the basic colors from the top row. The lower row shows several of the colors mixed with grays. To extend the color range even further, mix the colors from the center row with grays. You can either use warm or cool grays in your basic palette—I have never found it necessary to use the full range of grays available, although you may feel the addition of Nos. 1, 4, 6, and 8 grays will extend your color range.

In addition to the basic palette you may want to add a few special colors. Lemon yellow, pink, violet, peacock blue, and lime-green are colors I use occasionally. Check a color chart to see the complete range of colors available.

As an exercise, see how many different colors you can mix by using different colors over one another. Then try the same thing using colors and grays. When using markers over one another, you will have to clean the nib—just wipe the nib on a scrap sheet of paper until the other color is wiped off. As you develop, it would be a good idea to occasionally change your color palette, especially if you feel your paintings are looking too much the same—you will also learn a lot about color by changing your basic palette every once in a while.

Vermilion	Flesh
Geranium	Pale Sepia
Crimson	Lemon Yellow
Pale Rose	Bright Green

Pale Blue	Blue Green
Mariner Blue	Forest Green
Teal Blue	Nile Green
Aqua	Pale Olive

Mustard	No. 5 Gray
Putty	No. 7 Gray
No. 2 Gray	No. 9 Gray
No. 3 Gray	Black

Putty Flesh	Putty Pale Blue
Putty Lemon Yellow	Putty Geranium
Putty Bright Green	Flesh Lemon Yellow
Putty Pale Rose	Flesh Pale Olive

Flesh Aqua	Bright Green Pale Rose
Flesh Pale Blue	Bright Green Pale Blue
Pale Blue Pale Rose	Bright Green Aqua
Pale Blue Geranium	Lemon Yellow Pale Olive

Lemon Yellow Pale Blue	Pale Blue Crimson
Bright Green Geranium	Mariner Blue Vermilion
Vermilion Pale Blue	Mariner Blue Crimson
Vermilion Pale Olive	Geranium Nile Green

Flesh No. 2 Warm Gray	Pale Rose No. 7 Warm Gray
Flesh No. 4 Cool Gray	Geranium No. 2 Cool Gray
Flesh No. 5 Warm Gray	Geranium No. 4 Cool Gray
Pale Rose No. 4 Warm Gray	Vermilion No. 5 Cool Gray

Pale Blue No. 2 Cool Gray	Lemon Yellow No. 2 Warm Gray
Pale Blue No. 4 Cool Gray	Bright Green No. 2 Cool Gray
Aqua No. 2 Cool Gray	Bright Green No. 4 Cool Gray
Aqua No. 4 Cool Gray	Pale Olive No. 2 Cool Gray

Pale Olive No. 4 Cool Gray	Nile Green No. 4 Cool Gray
Lemon Yellow No. 4 Cool Gray	Pale Sepia No. 4 Cool Gray
Forest Green No. 4 Cool Gray	Pale Sepia No. 7 Warm Gray
Forest Green No. 7 Warm Gray	Vermilion No. 7 Warm Gray

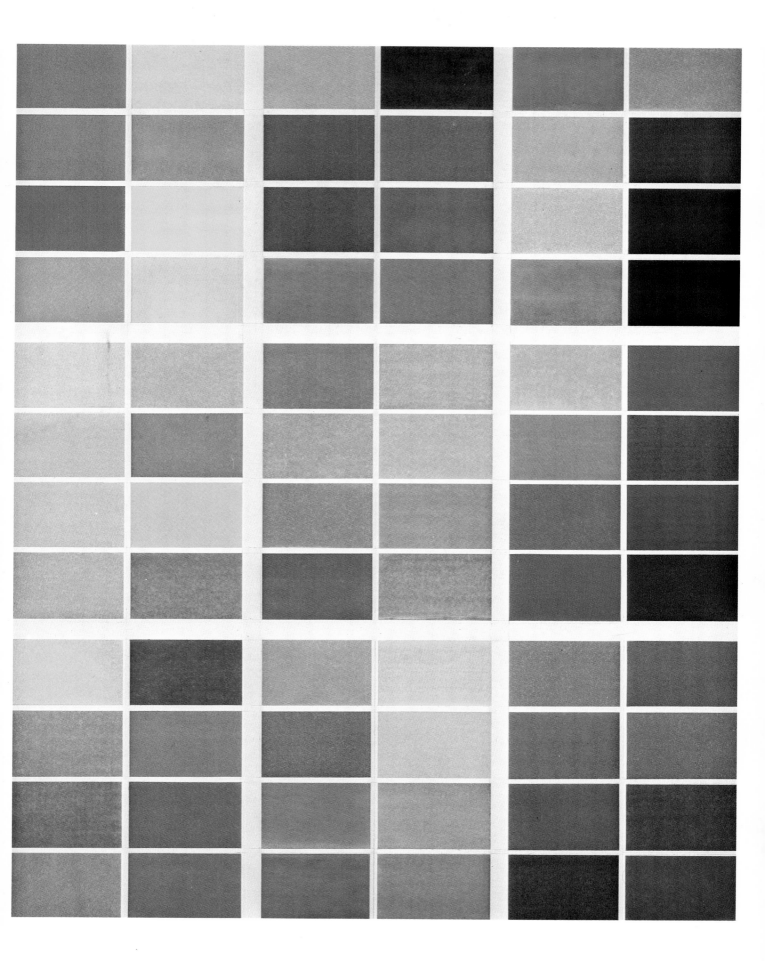

113

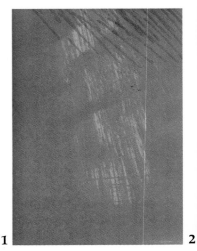

1

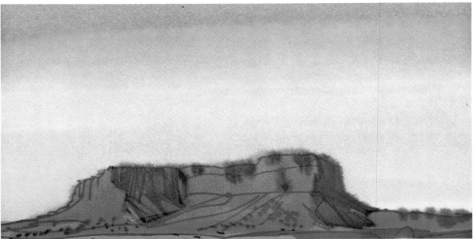

2

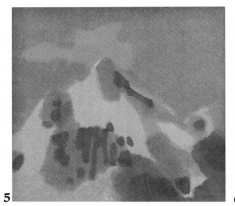

3

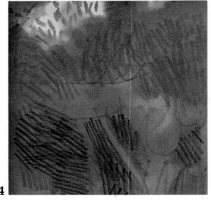

4

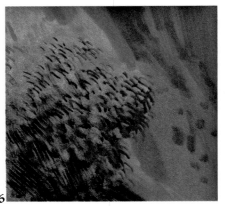

5

6

1. *A pale sepia background with a Nile green marker.*

2. *Solvents can help achieve soft and blended effects. Here the Bristol board was first dampened with a wash of Flomaster cleanser.*

3. *Shadows: teal blue on the barn; mariner blue on the tree; No. 2 gray with lilac on the silo.*

4. *I worked over the background shadow tones many times, using several colors under colored pencils.*

5. *The sky is pale rose, covered with pale sepia. For a sunlit glow on the snow, I used a flesh marker over the whole scene.*

6. *To coordinate the color in this scene, I used pale sepia over the whole picture after it was finished.*

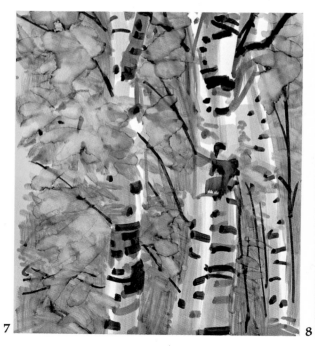

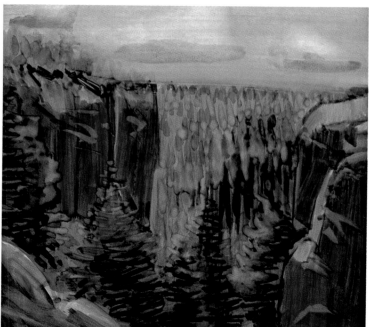

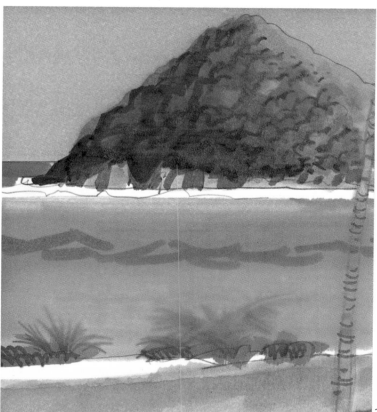

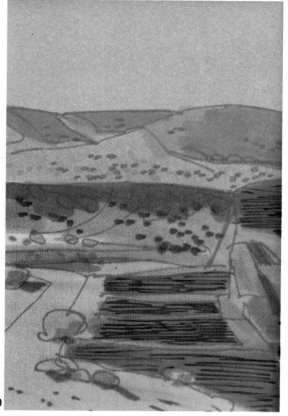

7. These birch trees were done on a sheet of coated paper—the dye colors don't soak in much on coated paper as they do on other papers. This enables areas to be reworked easily.

8. Another example done on coated paper. I cut back into the trees and cliffs with lighter colors to create more form and to highlight areas.

9. This example shows how well colors can be blended on a plate-finish Bristol, such as Aquabee. The water was created by using aqua over a pale blue, working quickly while the paper was still damp to assure a smooth blending of tone.

10. To create depth in this painting, I used cool colors in the background and warm colors in the foreground.

COLOR DEMONSTRATION 1. MICHIGAN FARM: BRISTOL

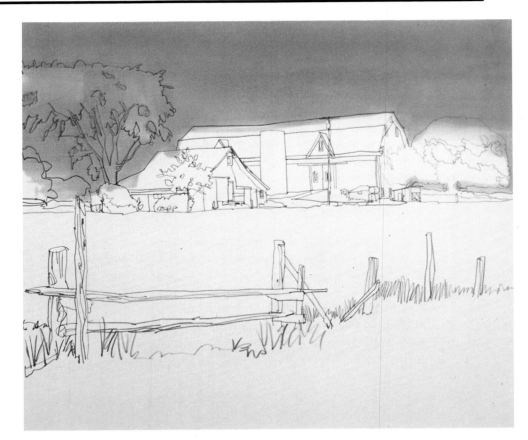

Step 1. *I start by doing a drawing of the scene with an HB grade graphite pencil on a plate-finish Bristol. This surface is excellent for pencil drawing, as it is very smooth. I add the sky with a pale blue Magic Marker, using the inner fiber core as shown in Demonstration 11. This method insures a smooth, flat sky tone.*

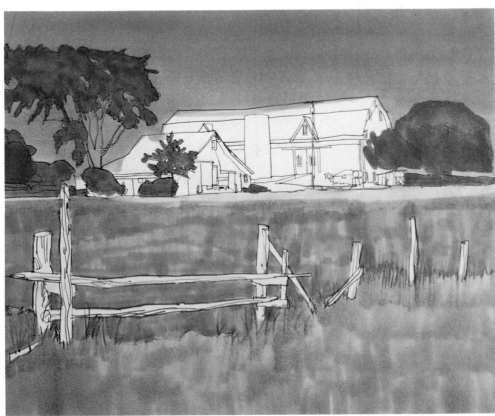

Step 2. *I work on the background field with green bice, and then use yellow green on the closer section. The foreground is put in with a mustard marker. Over the trees, I paint Spanish olive. At this point, I am covering up the white paper surface so I can establish my values and tones more easily. Never finish only one section of a painting—always gradually build up the whole picture.*

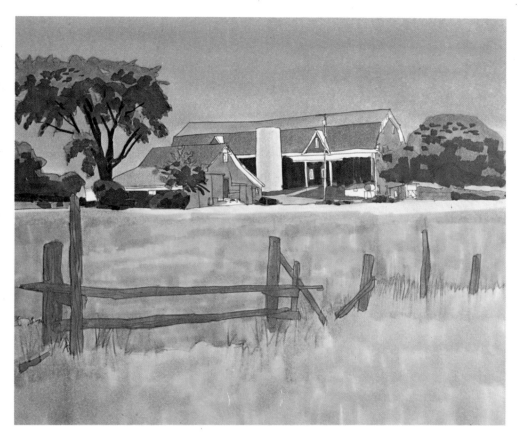

Step 3. *I add Nos. 2 and 5 cool gray markers to the roofs of the barn and the other building. On the sunny side of the barn, I use poppy, and on the shadow side, crimson. Nile green is used over the crimson to darken the shadow area, and the same green is also used on the trees. A No. 4 gray is put on the fence posts in the foreground, and the shadow areas on the trees are added with blue green.*

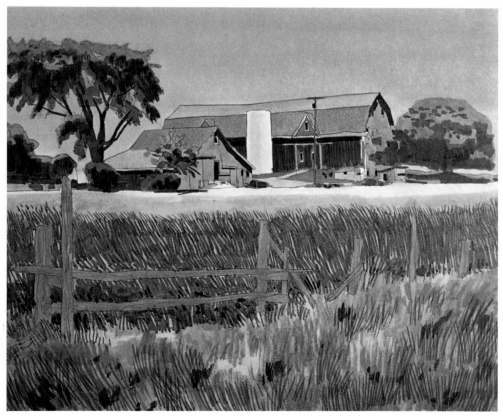

Step 4. *After I add Prussian blue shadows under the trees, I accent the roofs with black shadows. By using a Prussian blue marker with a rather dry nib, I am able to indicate a nice wood texture on the side of the barn. With a flagstone green, I render the grass texture in the middle field area. In the foreground, I add light suntan and bark, using strokes that help to create the illusion of grass. I add a pale sepia over the whole foreground to warm the color and also put a few darker patches in the grass.*

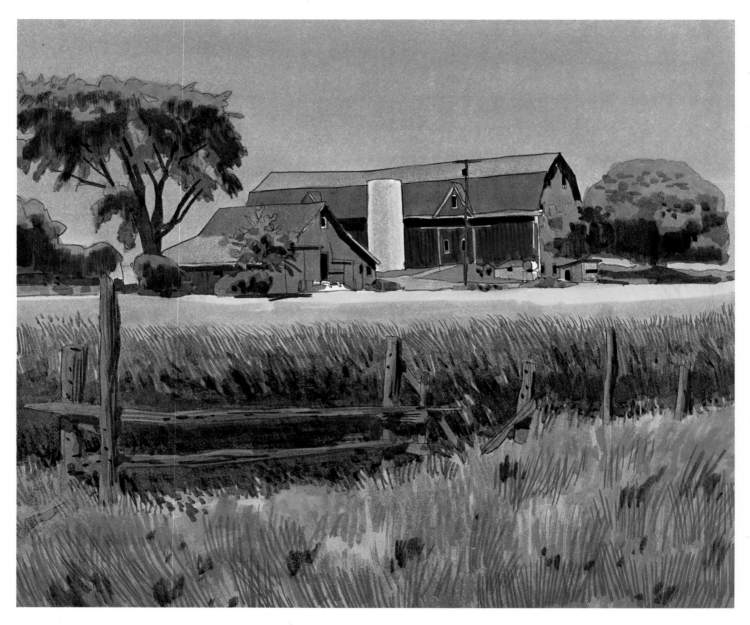

Step 5. *With a No. 7 gray, I slowly build up the foreground fence tones. On most paper surfaces, it's impossible to lighten tones, so it's best to build up your values gradually and avoid having them get too dark. With a No. 9 gray, I add accents to the fence to bring it out of the background. As a finishing touch, I use a No. 5 gray to separate the barn roofs more accurately.*

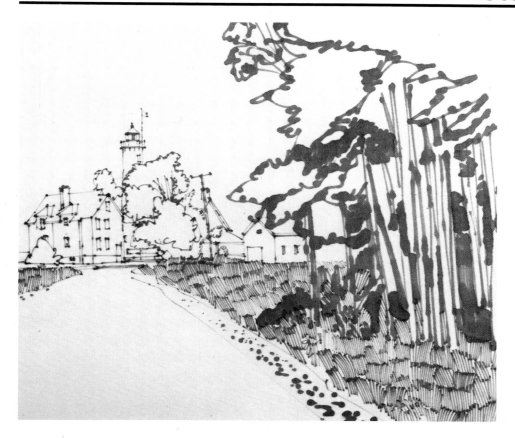

Step 1. *I begin by doing a drawing of the foreground trees with a No. 7 gray marker. Then I use a Pantone 417F to draw the buildings and the foreground grass texture. The stones at the road edge are indicated with the No. 7 gray marker.*

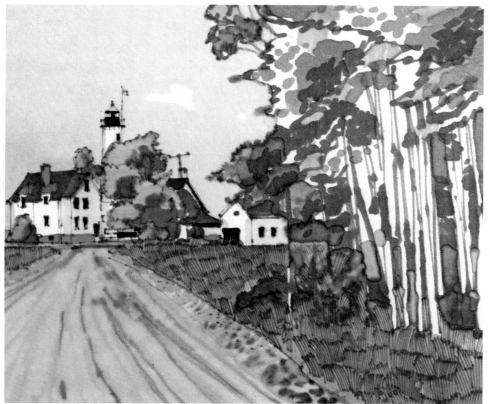

Step 2. *I use a yellow-green on the field and add mustard over this to warm up the color. I start to render the trees with a Spanish olive. Note that marker colors tend to appear darker on rice paper because the dyes saturate the paper. When first working with an unfamiliar paper surface, try a few colors on a piece of scrap paper to see how the colors go on.*

The sky is put in with a No. 1 warm gray Magic Marker, over which I use a frost-blue AD Marker.

Step 3. *On the road, I use a bright ivy AD Marker and add an indication of wheel tracks with a dark tan Magic Marker. On the side of the road, I use a light sand, and then I brush some of this color over the road. I use a Nile green and pale olive on the trees. On the background tree, I first use a Nile green, and then go over this with a green bice to brighten the color. I work a little more on the background tree with a pale blue and warm this by putting mustard over.*

At this point, I add mustard to the side of the road and a light warm gray to form a shadow on the buildings. Light bark is used on the roofs; the brick areas are put in with poppy. The windows and doors are accented with a Markette Thinrite black pen.

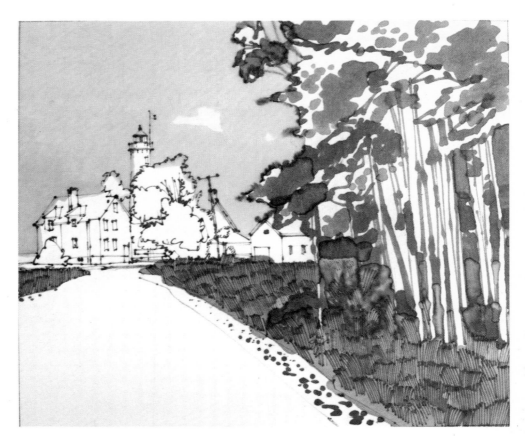

Step 4. *I add a pine-tree green to the shadow parts of the foliage and black to accent the trunks of the birch trees. The picture is shaping up nicely now. With a mariner blue, I put a few darks in the field and some shadows at the edge of the road.*

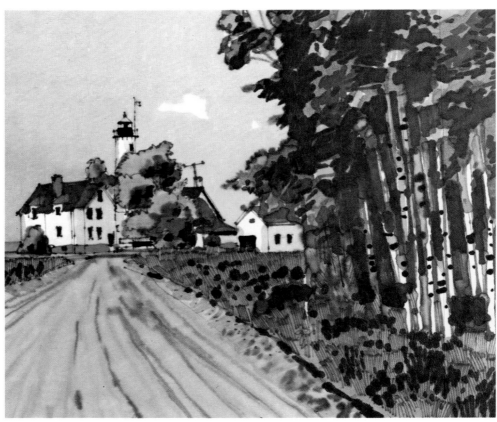

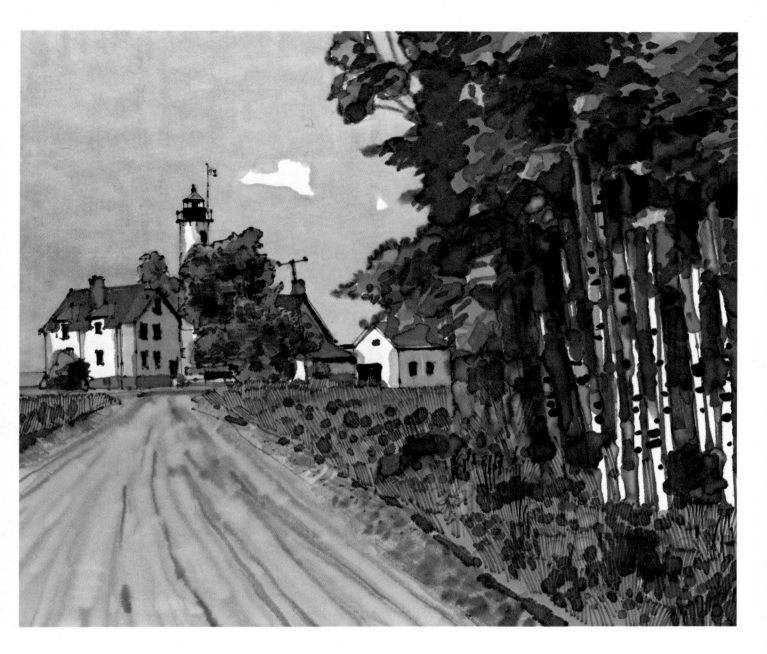

Step 5. *I add more dark areas to the trees with the mariner blue and black and put a few flowers in the foreground with a vermilion marker. I tone down the bricks on the shadow side with a No. 3 gray, finishing up the painting.*

This painting is more of an impressionistic rendition of the scene than a realistic one. The technique looks very much like watercolor and in fact is similar to the way I paint with watercolors.

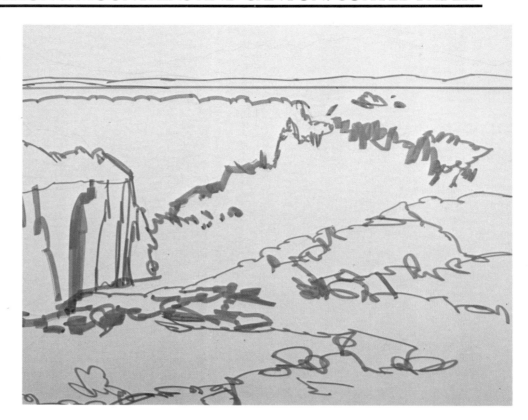

Step 1. *I do a drawing with a No. 7 gray marker. This drawing is simply a crude, but accurate, diagram of the scene.*

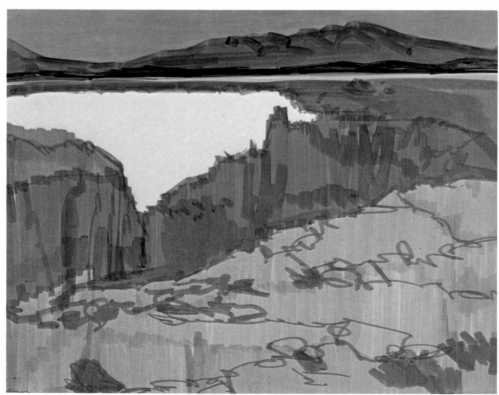

Step 2. *To put in the sky tone, I use a pale blue. The mountain in the background is done with a teal blue, using shadow accents of Prussian blue. Next, olive is added to the background, and a pale rose to the foreground. Then I start to put in the shadow area of the cliff with teal blue.*

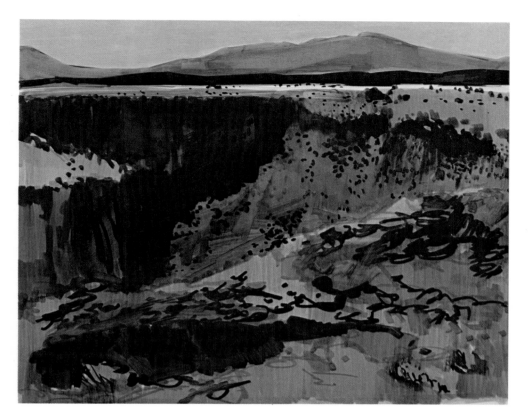

Step 3. *The shadow areas are completed, and then black is added to deepen them. I add a pale sepia and vermilion to the foreground area, and use black to put the rock textures and shadows over this.*

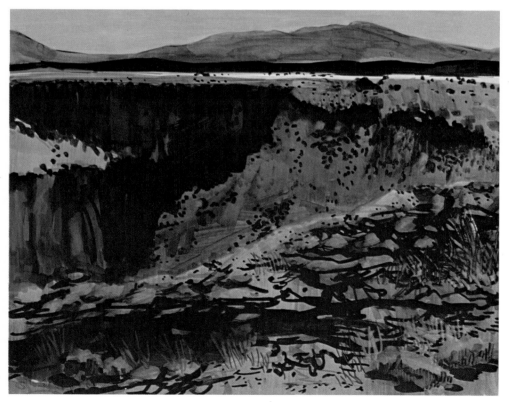

Step 4. *I continue to work on the foreground, adding more shapes and shadows with the black marker.*

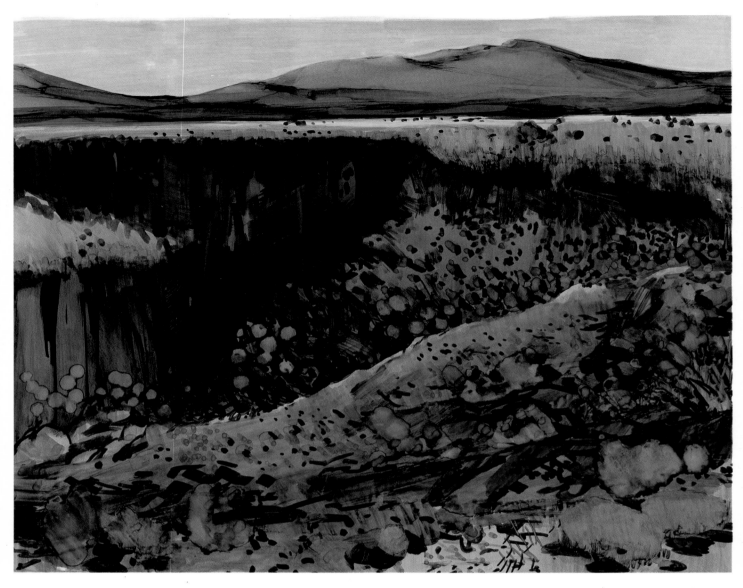

Step 5. *Dissatisfied with the foreground, I wash over the whole area with a paper towel and solvent. The Flo-master cleanser dissolves and blends the colors. I wash again over the area and lighten the colors considerably. When this is dry, I rework the whole foreground with vermilion, walnut, and black. The rocks in the canyon are done by using a light gray to cut back into the darker tone. I rework and lighten the mountain, creating more depth in the scene. Erin green is used over the olive to brighten the grass areas, and a flesh tone is put in the distant plain.*

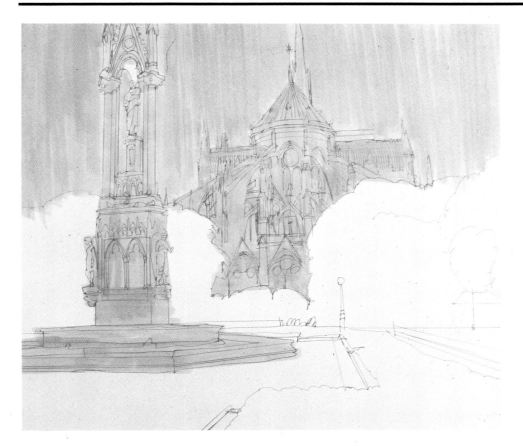

Step 1. *This painting is based on a 35mm color slide I took while vacationing in Paris. I start by first doing a basic drawing with an HB grade pencil on Kimdura, a synthetic plastic paper that takes pencil very well. I begin my color rendering by using a warm No. 4 gray over the building and foreground fountain. By working very quickly, I prevent the marker from dissolving my graphite pencil drawing. If you work over pencil too much or with a very wet marker, your drawing will be lost.*

The sky is roughly put in with a pale blue marker.

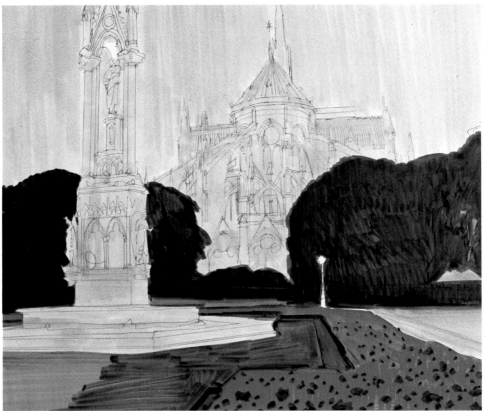

Step 2. *The flowers are put in using a crimson marker. I like to put in the brightest colors of a scene first, so I can judge how dark the other values should be. Then the grass is put in with a Nile green, which is quite bright—it will be toned down later. With a No. 9 gray, I underpaint the background trees. I will go over this tone later with lighter greens and a Prussian blue for the shadow tones. Next, I put in the shadow indications on the flowers with a No. 9 gray. Then I start to tone down the grass color with a teal blue.*

If I need to look at my color slide, I use a convenient daylight table viewer—they can be used with the lights on.

Step 3. *I use a pine-tree green over the trees—by using short strokes, I achieve a leaflike texture. On this type of paper, it's quite easy to cut back into dark tones and rework them with lighter markers, so I continue to add the green over the dark gray in the trees. I wasn't satisfied with how the grass was turning out, so with short, thin strokes I add a grass texture with pine-tree green. I cut back into the flowers with a vermilion to brighten them even more.*

With a No. 5 cool gray, I add an intermediate tone to the cathedral and fountain. With a No. 9 warm gray, I put in many of the building details. Then I use a mariner blue over the gray to achieve a cool cast to the shadow. Using a putty-colored marker, I highlight areas on the fountain and church. Next, with a forest green, I cut back into the trees to build up more form in this area, using strokes that simulate a leaf texture. Then I add black to the window and door areas.

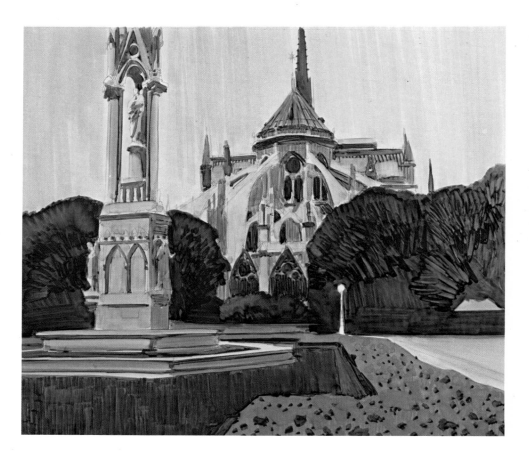

Step 4. *With a No. 1 gray marker, I cut back into the building, cleaning up edges and details. I do the same on the fountain in the foreground. The flowers are accented with cadmium red, and shadows are put in with forest green and black. Then I add a blue-green to the building shadows. The trees appear too dark, so I lighten them with a Spanish olive marker. (When working over a dark color with a lighter one, you may find that the nib becomes discolored—just rub it on a clean sheet of paper until it's clean.) Then I add a little more Nile green to the grass.*

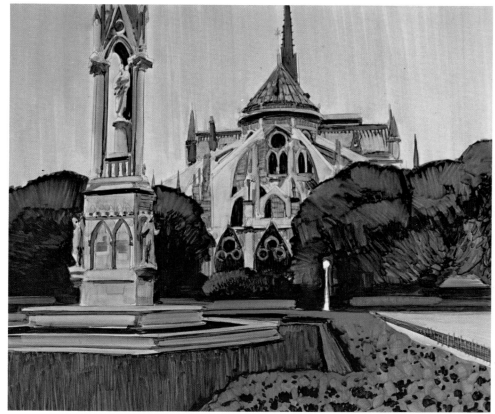

126

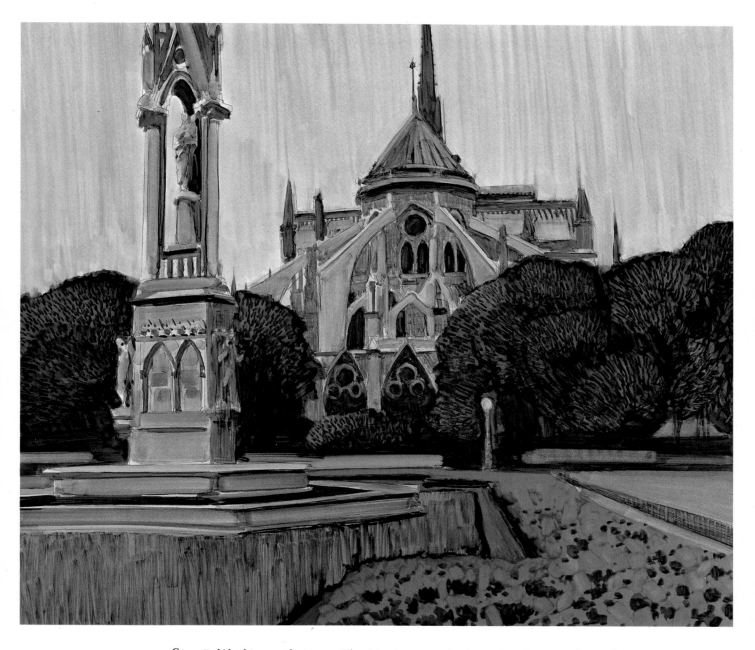

Step 5. *Working on the trees with a No. 9 gray and using a dotted texture, I tone down the area slightly. A light bark is used to warm the building and fountain. Now I feel the sky color should be better keyed to the rest of the painting, and add putty over the whole area.*

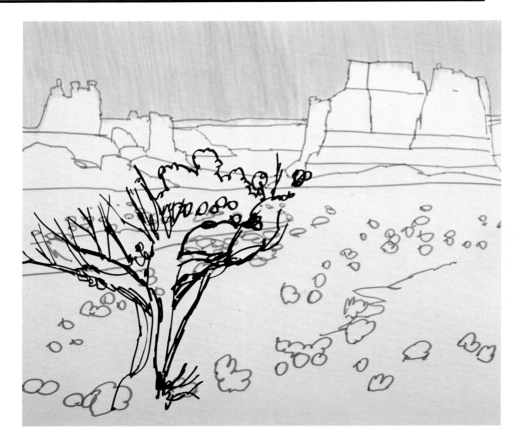

Step 1. *I do a basic diagram of the scene with a No. 7 gray marker. The foreground tree is drawn in with a black marker and the sky tone with first a warm No. 3 gray and then putty.*

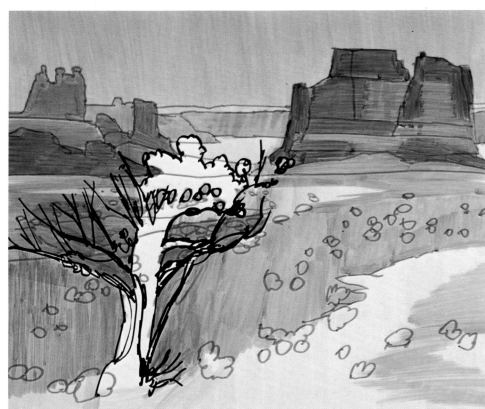

Step 2. *I cover most of the scene with a flesh tone. Then, on the background hills, I use a No. 5 gray and cut back in with a pale rose. I add light bark and suntan over the buttes. Light suntan is also used in the foreground area.*

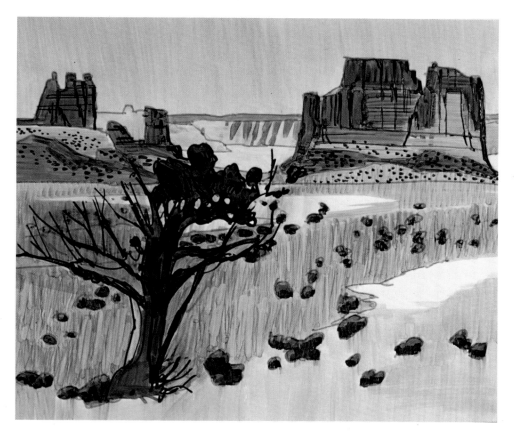

Step 3. *I add a pale rose over the whole foreground area and use a dark No. 9 gray to paint in some of the foliage. Then I darken the buttes with a No. 7 gray, adding surface detail, such as crevices and rocks. In the sunlit area in the background, I add barium yellow, warmed with a flesh color.*

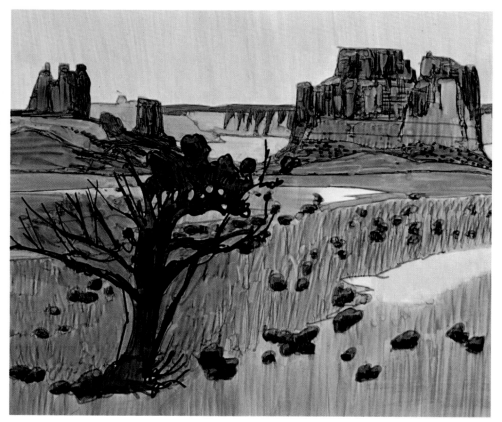

Step 4. *I use a shocking pink to warm the background and brighten the middleground area with cadmium orange. A light suntan is used over this to help relate the color to the whole picture. Then I go over the buttes with geranium and warm up the foreground color with mustard. Some of the shadow areas in the buttes are worked over with a No. 7 cool gray.*

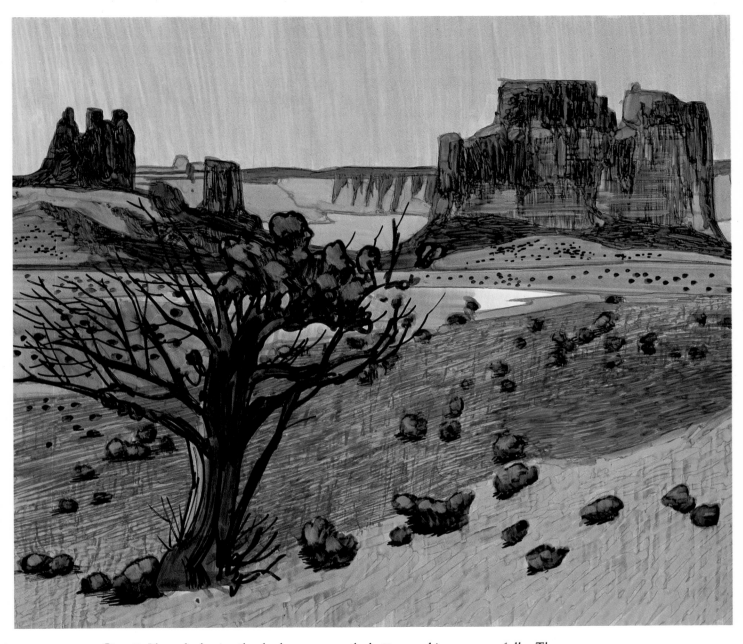

Step 5. *I keep darkening the shadow areas on the buttes, working very carefully. The texture in the middleground area is changed by using a mustard color with horizontal strokes. At this point, I decide to take out the pool of water on the right side of the picture. I darken the foreground with a walnut marker, and the painting is finished.*

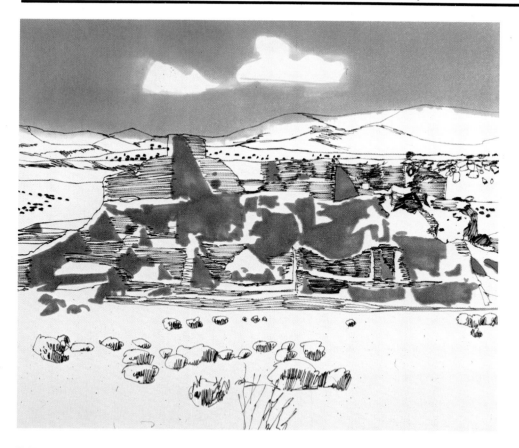

Step 1. *I do a drawing of the subject with a Niji Stylist pen, a very finely pointed marker pen, on a plate-finish Bristol. The very dark shadow tones are done with a No. 7 gray.*

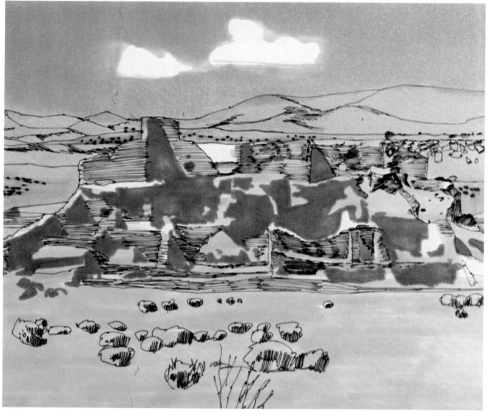

Step 2. *I use mustard and putty in the background, and, over the mustard, I put a flesh tone to warm the color slightly. I do the same thing in the foreground area, and then put a pale rose over the ruins.*

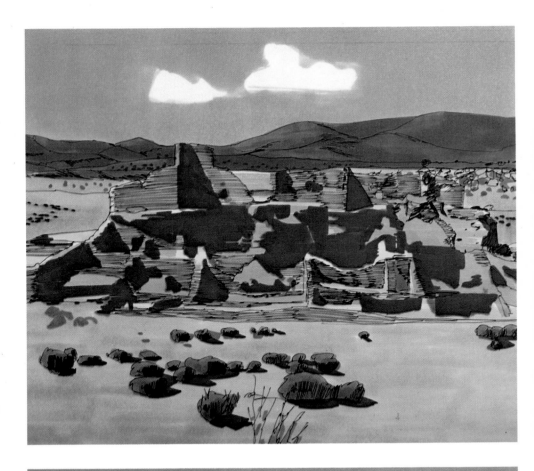

Step 3. *A pale olive is put on the foreground bushes, and mariner blue is used in the shadow portions. Then I use geranium over the ruins to warm them up—this exaggerates the color a bit. I will tone it down later with grays, leaving a little of the bright color in the sunlit areas. At this point, I put a very dark navy blue AD Marker into the shadow portions of the ruin. In the strong sunlight of the southwest, shadows appear to be deep blue—this tone will help achieve the overall sunlight effect I'm after in this scene. The distant hills are darkened with a teal blue and with No. 7 gray shadows.*

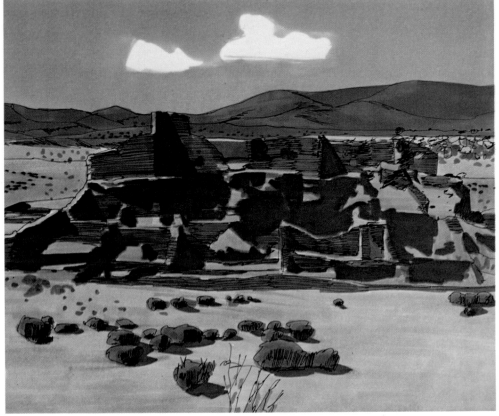

Step 4. *I put a pale rose over the background to relate the color to the overall tone a little better. Then I brighten some of the highlight areas on the ruin with a yellow ochre. Leather is used for the intermediate tones and over the deep blue shadows. This blends the color into the scene better, even though the blue in the shadows still dominates. I add an ochre color to the highlight areas on the ruin and also in the foreground foliage.*

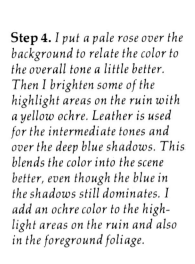

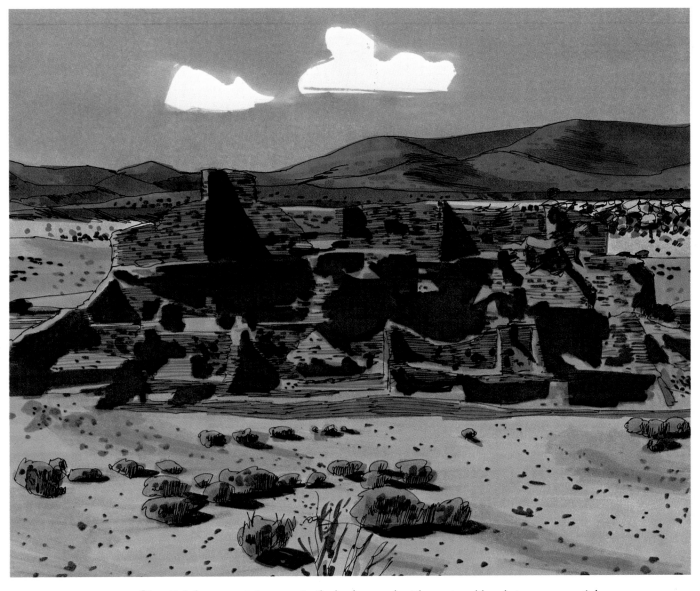

Step 5. *I deepen certain areas in the background with mariner blue, being very careful not to overwork them. Then I put a deep shadow into the background with Prussian blue. I use the Prussian blue also to add bricklike details to the intermediate tones on the ruin. A texture is put in the foreground area indicating stones and shadows, and a few grays are put in to suggest that the ground is uneven. Note that I did this painting from a 35mm color slide taken at Wupatki National Monument in Arizona.*

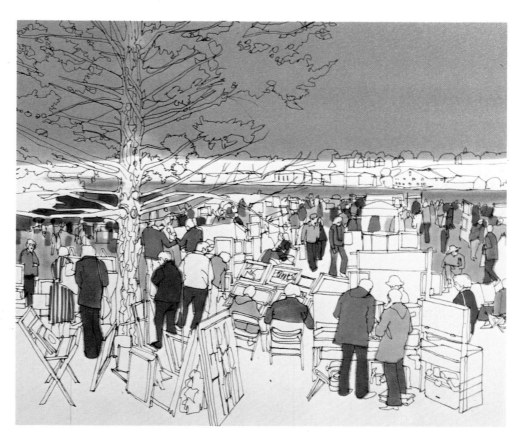

Step 1. *I start by doing a very detailed drawing of the scene with a Pilot Fineliner pen, an excellent pen that is perfect for drawing thin, even lines. The ink is water-soluble and, therefore, will not dissolve when markers are used over it. The sky is put in with a pale blue marker, using the fibrous core from inside the Magic Marker bottle. Most of the tones and colors can be put in this picture quite loosely, as the extensive linework tends to clarify the individual subjects.*

Step 2. *This was a very colorful scene, so I started putting in all the bright colors on the clothing. I am going to key the whole picture to these bright colors. Incidently, on the plate-finish Bristol, the marker colors soak in and thus appear a little darker than they would on a coated or synthetic paper. After blocking in the figures, I add a yellow-green to the grass.*

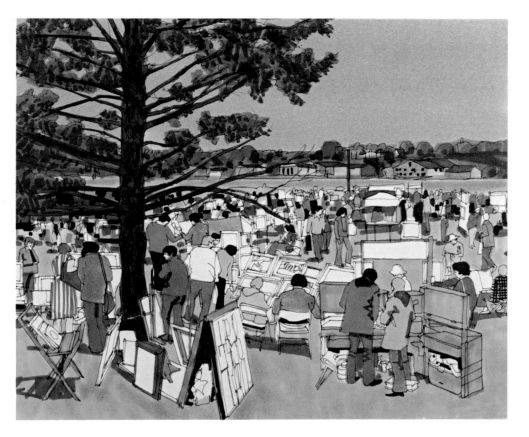

Step 3. I finish putting the grass in and add shadows of olive. Then I start to add a few blacks, so I have some darks to work against—it can be quite difficult to see the right values without these dark accents. Next, the foreground tree is put in with a forest green, and the trunk with a leather color. The distant trees are done using Spanish olive coated with Tahitian blue. Nos. 7 and 9 gray are used for bark and leaf detail in the tree—the No. 9 is also used to darken some of the background foliage. Continuing, I tone down some of the houses with putty and lime-green. A No. 5 shadow helps to define the buildings better.

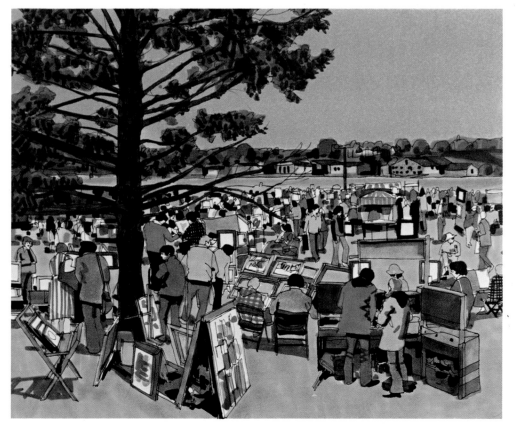

Step 4. I fill in many of the smaller areas and details. More darks are worked into the background to give the impression of detail. The painting is shaping up well at this point. I define the display on the right side by adding light bark as a shadow tone. Then I use a black Markette Thinrite pen to accentuate shoes, hair, and other details.

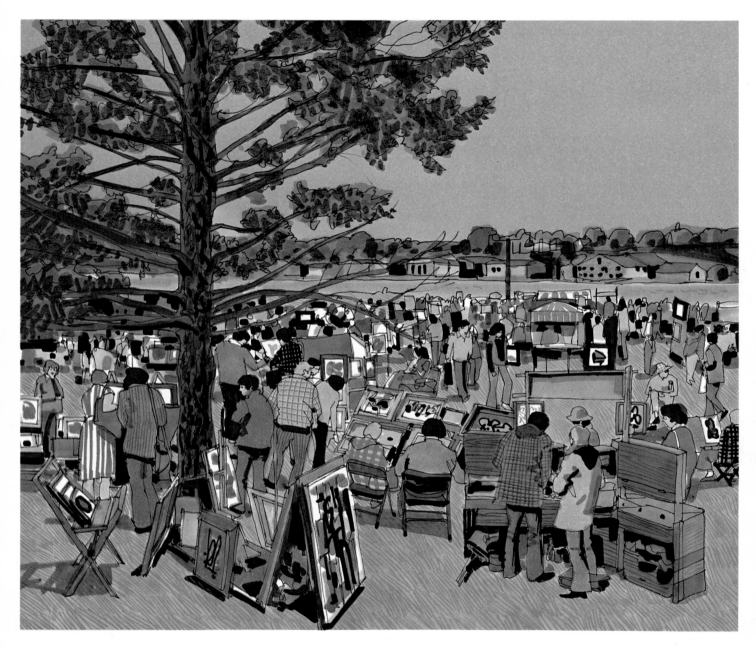

Step 5. *I continue to accent details throughout the picture with the black Markette pen. Color is put on the frames, paintings, and displays. I use a blue Prismacolor pencil to add texture to the grass. Colored pencils are also used on some of the clothing—these pencils work very well with markers. When using colored pencils over markers, be sure that the undercolor is very bright, as the pencils tend to darken and tone down the color.*

This technique is very similar to the one I generally use when doing advertising layouts and television storyboards. It is a fast, clean-looking technique that is well-suited for working under the pressure of a tight deadline.

CHAPTER TEN

Additional Hints

There are a few problems inherent in Magic Markers, as there are in any technique, but the advantages definitely outweigh them. Following are discussions of some problems and more suggestions.

THE PROBLEM OF FADING

Markers are dyes rather than pigments, and, in time, marker paintings will fade—especially if they are exposed to sunlight over a long period. Watercolor paintings have somewhat the same problem, but to a lesser degree. At this time, there is no remedy—hopefully in the near future there will be a solution to the problem of fading colors. Until a solution is found—and it may have been with the Steig Lightfast Watercolor Markers, a recent development—the real value of working in this medium is in the areas of drawing, sketching, doing preliminary color studies, and in the graphic arts. Advertising layouts and TV storyboards are not affected by the eventual fading of colors, and they are not meant to last permanently. Also, in both advertising and editorial art, almost immediate reproductions are made of illustrations, so fading is of no importance.

To minimize the problem, keep your work in a portfolio or frame them under glass. Don't hang anything in direct sunlight. Your paintings should certainly last as long as most watercolors, with a minimum of fading.

REPLENISHING OR ADDING NEW COLOR

To perk up a drying Magic Maker, just remove the cap from the container, pour in a little Flo-master cleanser (solvent), and put a few drops on the nib. This should put the marker in working order again.

If you want to, you can mix your own color for refilling a used up Magic Marker. Of course, this works best if the original color in the marker was very light, such as a light gray or putty. Use any of the eight Flo-master color inks and solvent, and use a ceramic tray for mixing. Put the inner fibrous core of the Magic Marker in the well to soak up the color—it's best not to use too much ink, or the marker will tend to drip. Then re-insert the fibrous core into the container.

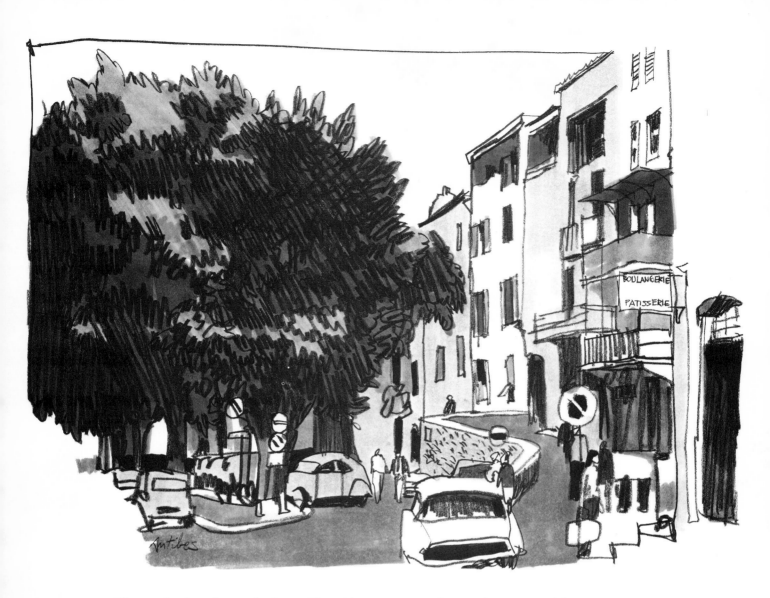

The underdrawing technique. *This technique is somewhat similar to some of the pencil and marker techniques shown in Chapter 2, but, in this case, a much more comprehensive drawing is done with more intermediate shading. After the drawing is lightly sprayed with a workable fixative at this intermediate stage, flat tones are put in. Other variations of this technique, such as underdrawing with ink in a drybrush technique or even using water-soluble markers, work very well. Some of these techniques are shown in the demonstrations.*

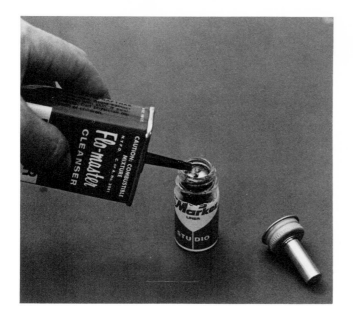

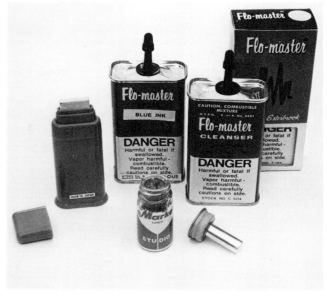

One of the advantages Magic Markers have over the other brands is that the top can easily be removed from the container. This means if you accidently leave the cap off and the nib of the marker dries, you can perk it up with a few drops of Flo-master cleanser. This should be put on the inside part of the nib as well as the outside. Frequently you can get a dried or almost empty Magic Marker going again by squirting some Flo-master cleanser on to the inner fibrous core.

Flo-master inks are available in several colors and come in a convenient can with a pouring spout. You can use these colors with the Flo-master felt pen or with a brush. Artist supply stores carry empty containers complete with felt nib, that can be filled with any mixture of dyes or inks.

EXPERIMENTING

Many interesting textures and effects can be created by using Flo-master colors with a crumpled paper towel and dabbing the color on the painting surface. You can also try spattering Flo-master colors or solvent by using an old toothbrush or dripping them on to the paper directly from the can. You can also blot the wet colors with another sheet of paper to see what textures occur. And, dyes can be combined with other drawing and painting materials not discussed in this book, such as crayons or opaque paint.

On occasion, I have even recut marker nibs to use for special effects. This can be done with a regular X-acto knife fitted with a No. 11 blade.

All of the above suggestions involve a little bit of a mess. To clean fingers, hands, or brushes that have been stained with Flo-master inks I always use the Flo-master cleanser. This solvent will also clean Magic Markers or other dyes from your hands. But be sure to use the cleanser in a well-ventilated room. It would be better not to get the dye on your hands in the first place, of course—if you can get used to working in rubber gloves, do so.

Don't worry about the mess, though, while you experiment—let yourself go, and you might come up with a very interesting rendering concept. Actually, this is the real fun of working with a new unfamiliar medium—to explore the possibilities. Experimentation with markers can result in most unusual effects, impossible to achieve with other painting mediums.

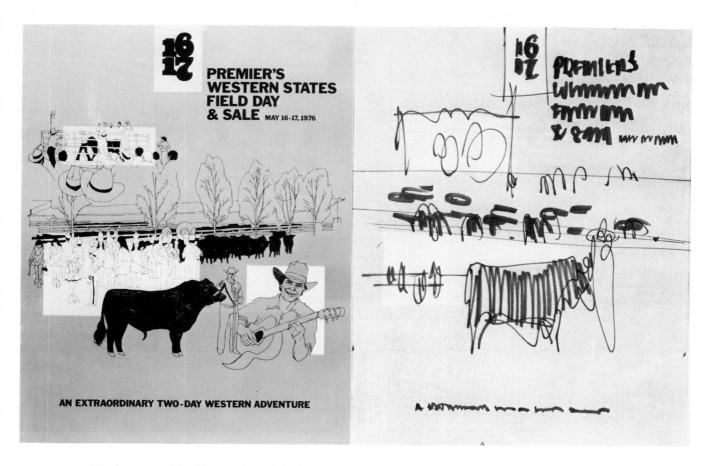

Markers used in illustration. *Markers offer a perfect solution when quick visual idea sketches are needed for ads, brochures, and TV storyboards. On the right is an example of a very rough layout done very quickly to show my client what I thought would work well for a proposed brochure cover. You can see how closely the sketch was followed in the printed piece at left.*

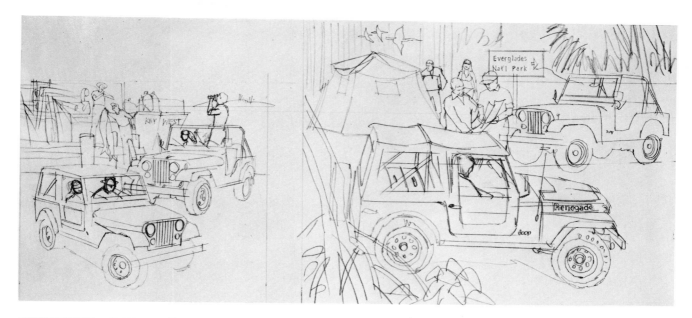

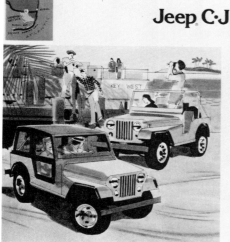

Jeep C·J

Pavli iovii iovii novocomensis in vitas cipum Praefatio, patere contendunt fa icecomivstatem nobilissimae Vicoc ta Romanorv Caesrrum oringe, Longb patere contendunt fabulosi penevnt itum famautem recentiora illustriorac cotentique enimae insgni memoria cum laude rei militaris, ciuilisque prud uerant, inuoluere videntur novocome imar ncidit Galuanius in id tempus quo est vir summa rerum gestarum gloria memorabilis. Captus enimiocum trium itur: sed non multo post carceris ca semel caesis Barabaris, vitus inuiras. Praefatit hic eximia ales ferunti Othoni gnitudeinesque animi, ca nente illo um in Syriam contendit, communicati iermo Montis ferrati regulo, qui a pro tur. Voluntariorvm enim equitum ac pe cipumavii iovii novocomensis in Vitas est vir summa rerum gestarum glori memorabilis. Captus enimtenad trium itur: sed non multo post carceris cater est vir summa rerum gestarum gloria memorabilis. Captus enimquiad trium itur: sed non multo post carceris cater semel caesis Barabaris, vitus inurias. zvli iovii novocomensis in vitat duodec gnitudeinesque animi, ca nente illo um in Syriam contendit, communicatis iermo Montis ferrati regulo, qui a pro tur. Voluntariorum enim equitum ac ped stemmat autem recentiora illustrora patern cidit Galuanius in id tempus qu est vir summa rerum gestarum gloria memorabilis. Captus enimiosius trium itur: sed non multo post carceris cater semel caesis Barabaris, vitus iniuria Caesrruit hic familiae qui ambit Othoni gnitudeinesque animi, ca nente illo um in Syriam contendit, communicatis iermo Montis ferrati regulo, qui a pro tur. Voluntariorum enim-equitum ac pe

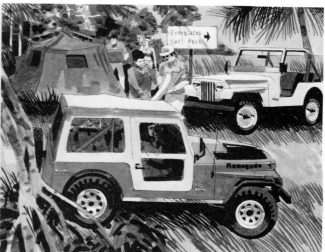

Jeep Catalog layout *An example of a comprehensive layout done for the Wayne Alexander Company, an advertising agency. At the top is the pencil sketch that was used as an underlay for doing the final rendering on layout paper. The tissue pencil drawing was positioned under a sheet of layout paper and traced through with a technical pen. Then markers were used to put in the tones.*

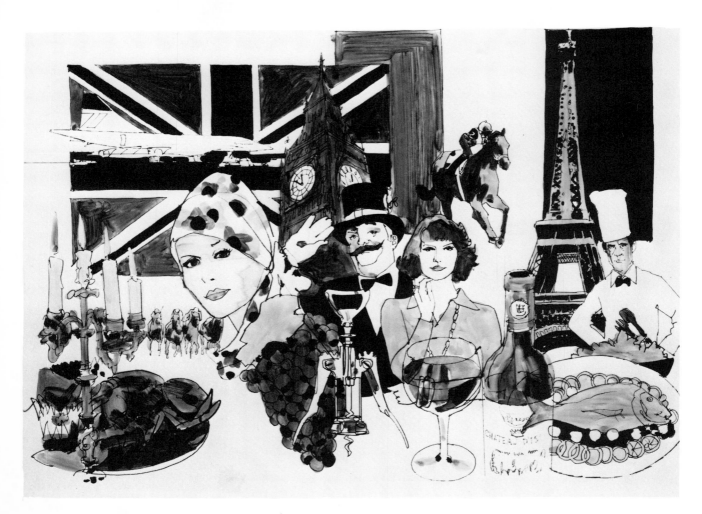

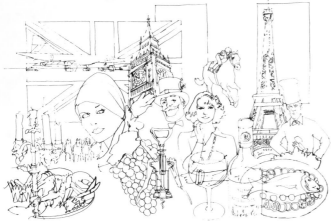

Another advertising layout. *In the advertising business an artist is usually up against a tight deadline, forcing the development of short-cut methods of working. The example here, done for David Gordon Associates of New York, was part of a very rushed job. I first did a very detailed pencil drawing on illustration board, and then photostated it down to the final printed size. Then I worked directly on the photostat with markers, completing my sketch. This is a very fast method of comprehensive layout illustrations. If the sketch is approved, you already have your pencil drawing on the illustration board ready to paint.*

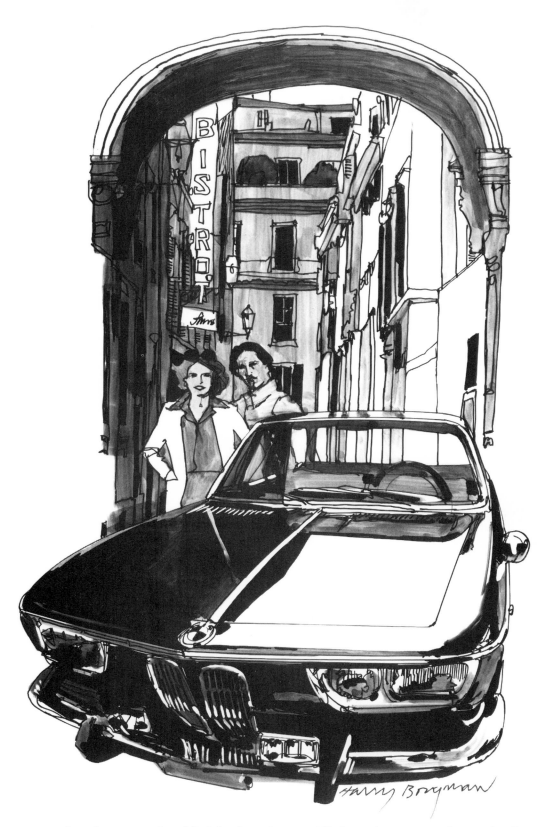

Another example of finished marker art. *The basic drawing was done with a Design Art marker 229 LU, a very finely pointed pen that works well on most surfaces, on a coated paper stock. The ink tends to soak well into the paper surface and will not dissolve when markers are used over it for tones. A very clean, fast technique that can be used for many subjects, whether you are doing an illustration or a painting.*

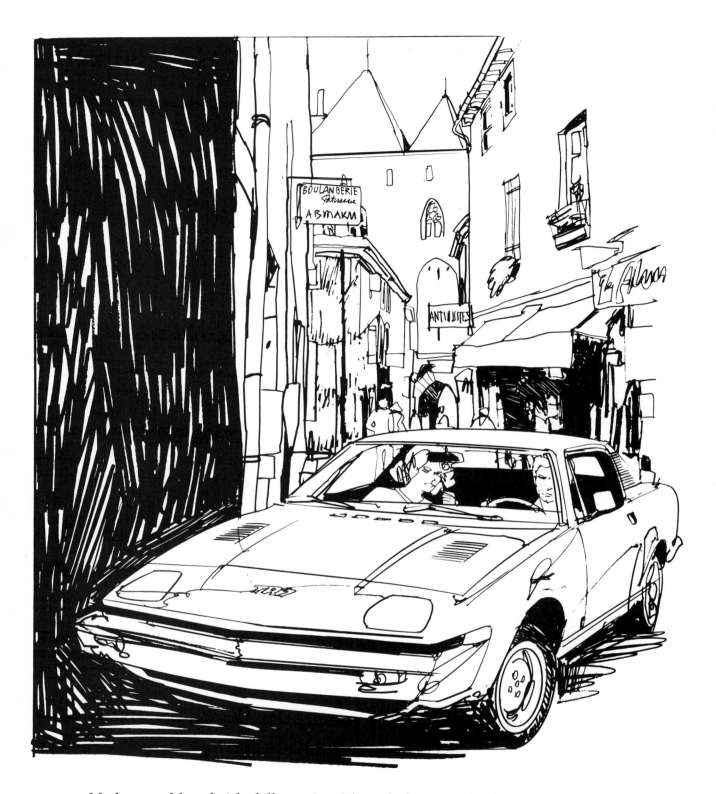

Markers used for a finished illustration. *I do a tight drawing with a Grumbacher Gamma all surface pencil on Kimdura, a plastic paper, following a rough pencil sketch. I then render markers directly over the pencil drawing, completing the illustration (opposite page). Notice that in certain areas the markers have dissolved the pencil lines, creating an interesting effect. With this technique you must work rather quickly—yet carefully—so you don't dissolve all your pencil lines. However, if some of the important lines are lost, they can easily be drawn back in with the pencil.*

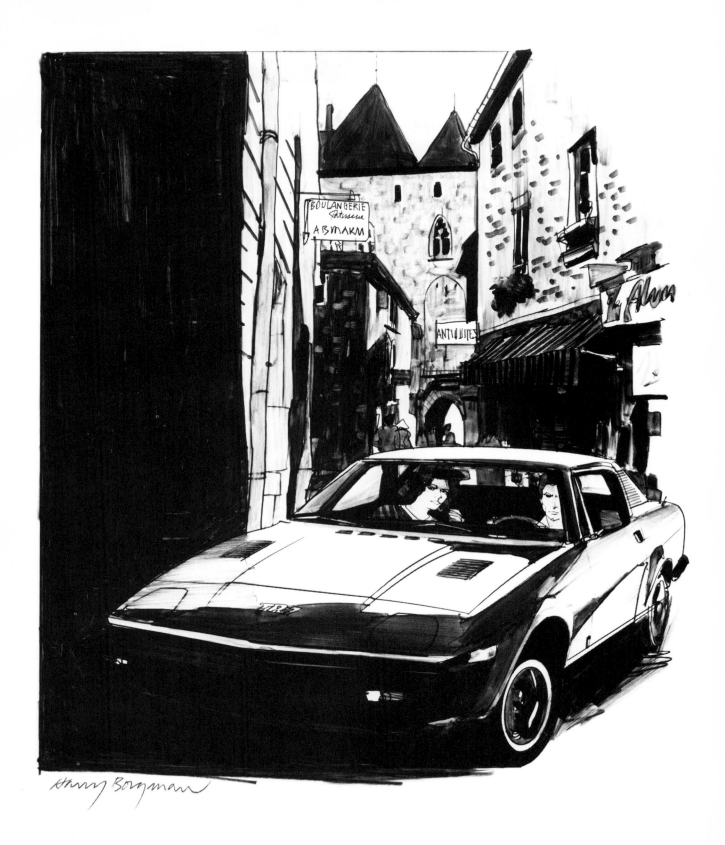

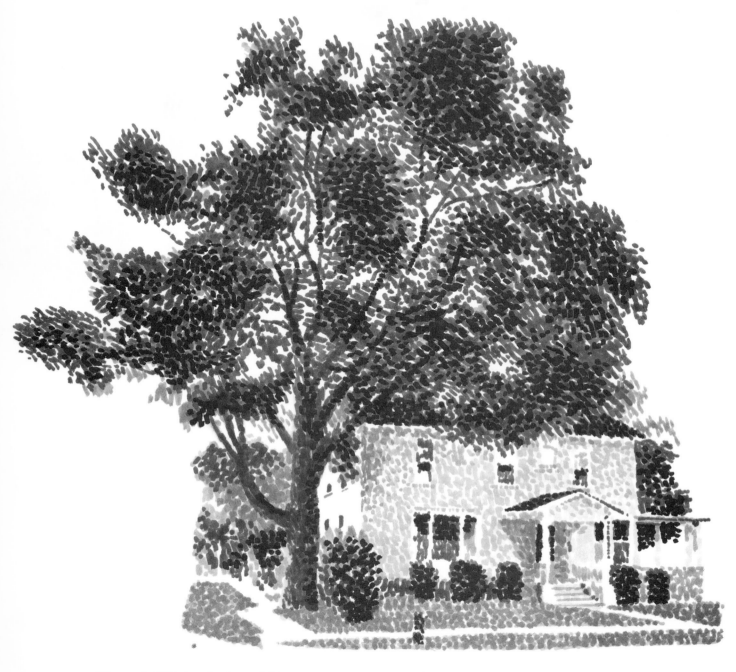

The pointillist technique. *This is a very interesting marker technique to experiment with. This painting was done on a plate-finish Bristol board.*

Bibliography

Ballinger, Harry R. *Painting Landscapes.* New York: Watson-Guptill, 1965.

Caddell, Foster. *Keys to Successful Landscape Painting.* New York: Watson-Guptill, 1976.

Curtis, Roger W., ed. Charles Movalli. *Color in Outdoor Painting.* New York: Watson-Guptill, 1977

De Reyna, Rudy. *Magic Realist Landscape Painting.* New York: Watson-Guptill, 1976.

Fawcett, Robert. *On the Art of Drawing.* New York: Watson, 1977.

Pitz, Henry C. *How to Draw Trees.* New York: Watson-Guptill, 1972.

Welling, Richard. *Drawing with Markers.* New York: Watson-Guptill, 1974.

Index